O P M L

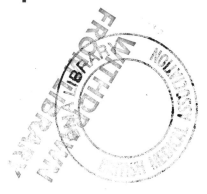

OXFORD PAIN MANAGEMENT LIBRARY

Pain in Older People

O P M L

OXFORD PAIN MANAGEMENT LIBRARY

Pain in Older People

Edited by

Peter Crome
Professor of Geriatric Medicine, Keele University, UK

Chris J. Main
Professor of Clinical Psychology,
Keele University, UK

and

Frank Lally
Research Fellow, Keele University, UK

OXFORD
UNIVERSITY PRESS

OXFORD
UNIVERSITY PRESS

Great Clarendon Street, Oxford OX2 6DP
United Kingdom

Oxford University Press is a department of the University of Oxford.
It furthers the University's objective of excellence in research, scholarship,
and education by publishing worldwide. Oxford is a registered trade mark of
Oxford University Press in the UK and in certain other countries

Reprinted 2013

British Library Cataloguing in Publication Data
Data available

Library of Congress Cataloging in Publication Data
Data available

ISBN 978-0-19-921261-3

Contents

Contributors

Panos Barlas
Research Fellow
School of Health and Rehabilitation,
Keele University,
Staffordshire, UK

Lisa Beeston
Senior Lecturer
Faculty of Health,
Staffordshire University,
Stafford, Staffordshire, UK

Dee Burrows
Consultant Nurse
Pain Consultants, Bullrush House, Great Missenden,
Bucks, UK

Jill Chanter
Senior Occupational Therapist
Chronic Pain Team,
Northern General Hospital,
Sheffield, UK

S. José Closs
Professor of Nursing Research
School of Healthcare,
University of Leeds,
Leeds, Yorkshire, UK

Claire Craig
Senior lecturer and researcher
Faculty of Health and Wellbring, Sheffield Hallam University, Sheffield, UK

Ilana B. Crome
Academic Director of Psychiatry and Professor of Addiction Psychiatry
Keele University Medical School, Harplands Hospital,
Stoke on Trent, Staffordshire, UK

Peter Crome
Professor of Geriatric Medicine
Keele University Medical School, Stoke on Trent,
Staffordshire, UK

Mark Deakin
Surgical Department,
University Hospital of North Staffordshire,
Stoke on Trent ,
Staffordshire, UK

Caitlyn Dowson
Consultant Rheumatologist
Rheumatology Dept.,
Haywood Hospital,
Stoke on Trent,
Staffordshire, UK

Kate M. Dunn
Lecturer in Epidemiology
Musculoskeletal Research Centre, Keele University,
Staffordshire, UK

Duncan Forsyth
Consultant Geriatrician
Addenbrooke's Hospital,
Cambridge, UK

Clare Jinks
Lecturer in Health Services Research, Musculoskeletal Research Centre,
Keele University,
Staffordshire, UK

Mike Jorsh
Academic Suite,
Harplands Hospital,
Stoke On Trent,
Staffordshire, UK

Francis J. Keefe
Pain Prevention and Treatment Research, Division of Medical Psychiatry, Duke University Medical Center, Durham, USA

Frank Lally
Research Fellow
Keele University Medical School, Stoke on Trent, Staffordshire, UK

Chris J. Main
Professor of Clinical Psychology, Calderbank Research Unit,
Keele University,
Manchester, UK

Andrew Moore
Department of Liaison Psychiatry,
Harplands Hospital,
Stoke On Trent,
Staffordshire, UK

Krishna Moorthy
Surgical Department,
University Hospital of North Staffordshire, Stoke on Trent, Staffordshire, UK

Bhanu Ramaswamy
Consultant Physiotherapist in Intermediate Care
Derbyshire County PCT,
Walton Hospital,
Chesterfield, UK

Elaine Thomas
Seniror Lecturer in Biostatistics
Musculoskeletal Research Centre, Keele University, Staffordshire, UK

Karen Walker-Bone
Senior Lecturer and Honorary Consultant in Rheumatology, Brighton & Sussex Medical School Education Centre, Princess Royal Hospital, West Sussex, UK

Sandra J. Waters
Assistant Professor
Pain Prevention and Treatment Research, Division of Medical Psychiatry, Duke University Medical Center,
Durham, USA

Preface

Pain is one of the commonest and most distressing symptoms of later life. It can affect patients' mood, quality of life, and independence. It may also adversely affect relationships and the health of carers. Until recently the whole subject of pain in older people has been relatively neglected both by practitioners and policy makers. The growing evidence base has allowed the production in both the USA and UK of guidelines on the assessment and management of pain in older people. We feel that it is timely to produce this introductory volume which we believe is the first on this subject in the UK. The authors are academics and practitioners and expert in their field. We have included chapters covering epidemiology, assessment, and common treatment modalities as well as individual chapters which deal with the most frequent causes of pain. Case histories have been used when appropriate to illustrate important clinical aspects. The important subjects of nursing, carers, and palliative care are also included. We hope that this book will provide a useful introduction on the subject for a wide multi-disciplinary readership working in both the primary health and social care areas as well as to undergraduate and postgraduate students in the health professions. The editors would like to express their thanks to all the authors for their contributions.

Peter Crome
Chris Main
Frank Lally

Keele, August 2006.

Introduction

Our intention in producing this pocket guide *Pain in Older People* has been to highlight this subject as a topic worthy of specific attention. During the last quarter of a century there have been significant advances in our understanding of the nature of pain and its management, but most research studies have not taken into account the special circumstances of pain management in older people. We believe that insufficient attention has been directed at this problem.

In our opinion, pain is often viewed from too narrow a biomedical perspective and in this volume we have wherever possible adopted a person-centred perspective based on a biopsychosocial model of illness, in which each of these components potentially impacts on the experience of pain.

We have attempted to represent pain as seen from a variety of perspectives and professional disciplines. We have tried to strike a balance between synthesis of the best available scientific evidence (particularly with regard to treatment and management) and offering specific advice on assessment and treatment for the practicing clinician.

We understand that ageing, in association with increasing rates of comorbidity offer a special challenge to clinicians, but we have been impressed with the richness and diversity of opinion which our colleagues have offered in their contribution to this volume.

We should like to finish on a note of optimism. In our view the treatment and management of pain in older people to date has been sub-optimal. We hope that this volume, in some small way, will stimulate reconsideration of the potential for new approaches to pain management in this most deserving group of patients and that our clinical colleagues will feel empowered to reconsider their clinical practice and further hone their skills within an evidence-based framework.

Peter Crome
Chris Main
Frank Lally

Keele, October 2006.

Chapter 1

The epidemiology of pain

Elaine Thomas, Kate Dunn, and Clare Jinks

Key points

- Pain is common in older adults and has a substantial multifaceted impact on both the individual and society.
- The majority of older adults experiencing pain do not seek the advice of health care professionals.
- There is a paucity of studies based solely in older adults.
- With the continued and projected growth of the aged population, pain and its effect on functioning and health care-seeking behaviour in older adults will become an even greater concern.

1.1 Introduction

The symptom of pain is of great clinical importance as it is often the complaint that motivates patients to seek health care. In recent years, pain has been seen as a problem on which clinicians and researchers can focus on in its own right, and not only as an expression of underlying pathology. With the continued and projected growth of the aged population, pain and its effect on functioning and health care-seeking behaviour in older adults will become an even greater concern (Badley & Crotty 1995). The specific area of pain in older adults is under-investigated, with few studies exclusively in older adults or with enough older adults to make robust estimates (Harris 2004). In addition, comparative estimates of the frequency of pain problems are sparse due to the lack of clear and consistent definitions of pain location, duration, and severity.

This chapter will review the current literature of the epidemiology of pain in older adults with specific focus on the size of the problem in the community and primary care, the commonest pain sites, the relationship with gender and age, and the multi-faceted impact of symptoms.

1.2 The size of the problem

Although much work in the field of pain research has been carried out in specialist pain clinics, the selectivity of the participants in this setting leads to questions about the wider applicability of the findings. To get a fuller picture of the burden of pain, researchers need to turn to the community and primary care.

Most of our current understanding of the epidemiology of pain comes from cross-sectional studies. Whilst these studies do provide useful data, they are limited in that they tell us about a single point in time. Information about the course of pain over time is needed to help determine the degree of persistence, the rate of the onset of new symptoms, and factors that can predict these patterns. Hence, prospective studies have an important role to play.

1.2.1 Community studies

The reporting of any pain in the older adult population is common, with estimates of 55–66% for 4-week prevalence (Scudds & Østbye 2001; Thomas *et al.* 2004) and 72–86% for annual prevalence (Brattberg *et al.* 1996; Brochet *et al.* 1998; Mobily *et al.* 1994) (Table 1.1). These figures are high but include pains that are transient in nature. When focusing on chronic pain, normally defined as symptoms lasting for more than 3 months, studies report prevalence estimates between 18–34% (Bowsher *et al.* 1991; Brochet *et al.* 1998). When examining the course of symptoms over time, it is clear that pain persists both in terms of any pain (Donald & Foy 2004) and chronic pain (Elliott *et al.* 2002).

The current evidence regarding gender differences suggests that females tend to be more likely to report pain than males. The evidence for a relationship with age is less clear; a review suggested a decrease in symptoms over the age of 60 years (Helme & Gibson 2001), but two large population-based studies report that the prevalence of pain remains constant with increasing age (Scudds & Østbye 2001; Thomas *et al.* 2004). A small number of studies have quantified the degree of pain and the common theme is that pain of a chronic, severe, or persistent nature appears to increase with age (Brattberg *et al.* 1996; Brochet *et al.* 1998; Mobily *et al.* 1994).

Measuring the socio-economic status of older people presents particular difficulties. However, studies that have examined the relationship between measures of social class and pain in older adults have shown a strong relationship with the higher reporting of pain in manual occupations (Saastamoinen *et al.* 2005).

Table 1.1 Period prevalence of pain in population-based studies exclusively in older adults

Study	Age (years)	Number in study	Period	Overall prevalence	Prevalence with age				
					50–59 yrs	60–69 yrs	70–79 yrs	80–89 yrs	90+ yrs
Scudds & Østby (2001)	70+	5700	4 weeks	55%			56%	56%	60%
Thomas *et al.* (2004)	50+	7878	4 weeks	66%		69%	63%	63%	63%
Brochet *et al.* (1998)	65+	741	12 months	72%		65%	64%	64%	74%
Brattberg *et al.* (1996)	77+	537	12 months	73%			75%	75%	68%
Mobily *et al.* (1994)	65+	3097	12 months	86%		88%	86%	86%	79%

1.2.2 **Primary care studies**

Although the population prevalence of pain is high, not everyone seeks health care for their symptoms. However, pain conditions are still one of the most common reasons for seeking primary health care, and represent a significant burden on health services. One recent study indicates that 10% and 12% of elderly men and women respectively seek treatment for neck pain, with 13% and 19% seeking treatment for back pain (Hartvigsen *et al.* 2006). Work from the UK indicates that 10% of older people consult a general practitioner with a new episode of knee pain each year (Jordan *et al.* 2006). These figures imply that between a fifth and a third of pain sufferers consult for their problem, a similar figure to that reported in working age populations, although one study of low back pain found that nearly 75% of sufferers consulted for their problems (Lavsky-Shulan *et al.* 1985).

Although there have been a range of studies of the prognosis of consulters with pain in primary care, no studies (as far as we are aware) have specifically focused on older people. As many of the prognostic factors are work-related (e.g. job satisfaction), and some conditions are less common and rarely studied in younger populations (e.g. knee pain), we probably cannot directly extrapolate findings from the current studies to older people. Some indicators of poor prognosis, such as poor psychological status, comorbidity, and duration of symptoms, are also likely to be relevant to some pain conditions in older populations, but more research is needed in this area.

1.3 Location of pain

In addition to the patterns with any pain, researchers have also examined the variation in prevalence across specific regional pain sites and the concept of widespread pain—the concomitant presentation of multiple regional pain syndromes—has also been studied as a specific entity.

1.3.1 **Regional pains**

This review will concentrate on the four pain sites most commonly reported in a recent, large population-based study of older adults; that is knee, hip, hand, and low back (Thomas *et al.* 2004). There are a number of other pain sites that are common in the community, for which there is limited information among older people, for example non-specific chest pain, neck pain, pelvic pain, and foot pain.

1.3.1.1 ***The knee and hip***

In older age groups, the knee is the most common site of regional pain (Thomas *et al.* 2004): UK population-based studies have estimated that between 28% and 47% of older adults have knee pain each year

(Jinks *et al.* 2004, O'Reilly *et al.* 1998). Similar prevalences across gender have been reported up to the age of 75 years. Symptoms are significantly more common in women (51%) than men (38%) in the oldest old (Jinks *et al.* 2004).

Approximately 25% of adults aged 50 and above reported recent hip pain in a UK population-based study (Thomas *et al.* 2004). Another UK study reported that 18% of adults aged 58 reported regular swelling, pain, or stiffness in their hips (Adamson *et al.* 2006). The relationship between hip pain and gender is not clear. For example, a Dutch study reported that 21% of women aged 65 and over had hip pain, with a lower estimate in men (11%) (Picavet & Schouten 2003). However, findings from another population study show a higher prevalence of hip pain in men than women in this age group (18% in men vs. 9% in women) (Birrell *et al.* 2005).

Prospective data on knee and hip pain in older adults are rare, and most studies have focused on radiographic changes rather than changes in pain and disability. Severity of symptoms and the total number of knee or hip joints with pain are associated with persistent knee or hip pain (Dawson *et al.* 2005). Although knee and hip symptoms frequently progress, 14% of older adults with both hip and knee pain will have resolved pain over a one-year period (Dawson *et al.* 2005). Female gender is not significantly associated with progression of knee pain in older adults (Dawson *et al.* 2005).

1.3.1.2 **The hand**

Interestingly, less research attention has been given to the hand despite it being one of the most common sites of pain and osteoarthritic change in this age group. Population-based studies have reported that up to 30% of older adults will have hand symptoms in a one-month period and that these symptoms are persistent and are strongly associated with severe disability (Dahaghin *et al.* 2005; Dziedzic *et al.* 2004). Moreover, severe hand pain and disability have been shown to increase with increasing age (Dziedzic *et al.* 2004).

1.3.1.3 **The low back**

Low back pain is common in all age groups, but some studies appear to show a fall in prevalence in those aged over 60 years, for example one UK study showed that prevalence was slightly higher in 45–59-year-olds compared with those aged 60+ (Papageourgiou *et al.* 1995). However, evidence is now emerging that there is not a straightforward pattern of low back pain with age (Dionne *et al.* 2006). The exact relationship may depend on symptom severity, and be related to the increasing prevalence of other comorbidities; older people may still have their back pain, but in the case of milder symptoms, they may no longer consider it to be an important problem, hence an apparent fall in reporting. Most studies in low back pain show that prevalence is higher in women than men, for example

44% and 35% respectively among people aged 60 years and older (Papageourgiou *et al.* 1995).

Few prospective studies have specifically investigated factors associated with back pain in older people, but cross-sectional studies indicate that around 25% of sufferers have difficulties performing their daily activities, and have highlighted associations of low back pain with psychological status, comorbidity and low physical activity (Cecchi *et al.* 2006; Hartvigsen *et al.* 2006).

1.3.2 **Widespread pain**

Pain symptoms often co-exist in the same patient, and it is difficult to disentangle whether they are separate conditions with different aetiology and prognosis, or whether they are part of a widespread pain syndrome. This is complicated by the fact that, for regional pains, presence of pain in other areas of the body is often an indicator for poor prognosis. But however we look at this, reporting of pain at a number of sites is common. In studies in the USA and Sweden, 59% and 47% respectively of the older population reported pain at multiple sites (Brattberg *et al.* 1996; Mobily *et al.* 1994), and a study in the Netherlands reported a point prevalence of pain in two or more sites of 28% and 46% among men and women respectively aged 65+ years (Picavet & Schouten, 2003).

1.4 **Impact**

The experience of pain at some point during life is almost inevitable, and hence may be perceived as part of normal life. However, the impact of symptoms on an individual's life can be substantial and multi-faceted, affecting areas such as function, social roles, and economics. Moreover, the effects of pain also have an impact at the societal level, in terms of the economy and health and social services.

1.4.1 **Economics**

Among populations of working age, around a quarter (for hip or knee pain) to a third (for low back pain) of sufferers take time off work because of their pain problem during a one-year period (Picavet & Schouten, 2003). There is little data specifically on older people, but it could be assumed that older people who were still in employment might experience rates of work absence similar to these. Given the high prevalence of pain conditions among older adults, the ageing population, and the increasing age of retirement, this represents a significant economic burden that could well increase in the future.

There is a lack of data about the costs of pain syndromes to the individual. A Canadian study found the average annual costs of hip and knee osteoarthritis to the individual adult (≥55 years) was $12,200

($CDN). Time lost from employment and leisure by individuals and their unpaid caregivers accounted for 80% of the total (Gupta *et al.* 2005). A UK study found that the median monthly spend on complementary medicines by adults aged 55 and over with knee osteoarthritis was £5.00 (range £0.66 to £150). Higher spending was linked to social class. The median spend on complementary therapists was £13.50 (range £1 to £150) (Jordan *et al.* 2004). Another population study in the UK found that less than 2% of the general older population used any private treatments or services for their knee pain (Jinks *et al.* 2004), but financial costs of these are not provided.

1.4.2 **Function**

Studies have consistently shown that a substantial proportion of older adults who experience pain also report associated difficulties in different aspects of life, including activity limitation, quality of life, pain interference, and participation. In contrast to the similar prevalence of pain across age groups, the impact of such symptoms has been shown to be related to age, with a pattern of increase from those aged 50–59 years through to those aged 80+ years (Thomas *et al.* 2004).

1.4.3 **Public health**

The high prevalence of pain in older people, its impact in terms of disability, and the existence of some modifiable risk factors means that identifying approaches to prevention is a public health priority. However, few studies have addressed this at the population level. Obesity is one obvious target for preventative activity.

Strategies to avoid excess weight, facilitate weight loss, and increase physical activity in older adults are under researched. A complex range of barriers exists which challenge the uptake of physical activity in the elderly. These include lack of social support, embarrassment, and confidence, poor general health, environmental factors, financial matters, lack of appropriate facilities, and lack of knowledge about the benefits of exercise. Pain conditions contribute significantly to poor quality of life and so reducing this burden will have substantial implications for the health of older people. Research needs to focus on testing and implementing public health interventions to achieve this.

Box 1.1 Facts

- Individuals with a body mass index >30 kg/m^2 have twice the odds of reporting hip pain and nearly two and a half times the odds of reporting knee pain. (Adamson *et al.* 2006)
- Prevalence of back pain in adults aged 60 and over increas according to weight (Andersen *et al.* 2003)
- In the US, the percentage of arthritis cases attributable increased from 3% to 18% between 1971 and 2002 (L 2005)

1.5 Conclusion

This review of available evidence of pain in older people has shown that despite growth in the size of the aged population, there is a paucity of research on pain focused specifically on this section of the population. We do know that pain is common in older adults and has a substantial impact on both the individual and society, and that most older adults with pain do not seek health care. Research should now focus on determining the longer term individual and public health consequences of pain with the aim of reducing this burden in the older population.

References

Adamson J, Ebrahim S, Dieppe P, *et al.* (2006). Prevalence and risk factors for joint pain among men and women in the West of Scotland Twenty-07 Study. *Ann Rheum Dis*, **65**, 520–4.

Andersen R, Crespo C, Bartlett S, *et al.* (2003). Relationship between body weight gain and significant knee hip and back pain in older Americans. *Obes Res*, **11**, 1159–62.

Badley EM and Crotty M (1995). An international comparison of the estimated effect of the aging of the population on the major cause of disablement, musculoskeletal disorders. *J Rheumatol*, **22**,1934–40.

Birrell F, Lunt M, Macfarlane G, *et al.* (2005). Association between pain in the hip region and radiographic changes in osteoarthritis: results from a population-based study. *Rheumatology*, **44**, 337–41.

Bowsher D, Rigge M, and Sopp L (1991). Prevalence of chronic pain in the British population: a telephone survey of 1037 households. *Pain Clinic*, **4**, 223–30.

Brattberg G, Parker MG, and Thorsland M (1996). The prevalence of pain among the oldest old in Sweden. *Pain*, **67**, 29–34.

Brochet B, Michel P, Barberger-Gateau P, *et al.* (1998). Population-based study of pain in elderly people: a descriptive survey. *Age Ageing*, **27**, 279–84.

Cecchi F, Debolini P, Lova RM, *et al.* (2006). Epidemiology of back pain in a representative cohort of Italian persons 65 years of age and older: the InCHIANTI Study. *Spine*, **31**, 149–55.

Dahaghin S, Bierma-Zeinstra SM, Reijman M, *et al.* (2005). Prevalence and determinants of one-month hand pain and hand related disability in the elderly (Rotterdam study). *Ann Rheum Dis*, **64**, 99–104.

Dawson J, Linsell L, Zondervan K, *et al.* (2005). Impact of persistent hip or knee pain on overall health status in elderly people: a longitudinal population study. *Arthritis Rheum*, **53**, 368–74.

Dionne CE, Dunn KM, and Croft PR (2006). Does back pain prevalence really decrease with increasing age? A systematic review. *Age Ageing*, **35**, 229–34.

Donald IP and Foy C (2004). A longitudinal study of joint pain in older people. *Rheumatology*, **43**, 1256–60.

Dziedzic K, Thomas E, Hill S, *et al.* (2004). MRC Hand programme–prevalence of hand problems and hand pain in older people: a survey of the general population in North Staffordshire. *Rheumatology*, **43**, 88.

Elliott AM, Smith BH, Hannaford PC, *et al.* (2002). The course of chronic pain in the community: results of a 4-year follow-up study. *Pain*, **99**, 299–307.

Gupta S, Hawker GA, Laporte A, *et al.* (2005). The economic burden of disabling hip and knee osteoarthritis (OA) from the perspective of individuals living with this condition. *Rheumatology*, **44**, 1531–7.

Harris L (2004). *Review of prevalence of pain in older adults.* MMedSci Thesis, Keele University.

Hartvigsen J, Frederiksen H, and Christensen K (2006). Back and neck pain in seniors–prevalence and impact. *Eur Spine J*, **15**, 802–6.

Helme RD, and Gibson SJ (2001). The epidemiology of pain in elderly people. *Clin Geriatric Med*, **17**, 433–56.

Jinks C, Jordan K, Ong BN, *et al.* (2004). A brief screening tool for knee pain in primary care (KNEST). 2. Results from a survey in the general population aged 50 and over. *Rheumatology*, **43**, 55–61.

Jordan K, Sawyer S, Coakley P, *et al.* (2004). The use of conventional and complementary treatments for knee osteoarthritis in the community. *Rheumatology*, **43,** 381–4.

Jordan K, Jinks C, and Croft P (2006). A prospective study of the consulting behaviour of older people with knee pain. *Br J Gen Pract*, **56**, 269–76.

Lavsky-Shulan M, Wallace RB, Kohout FJ, *et al.* (1985). Prevalence and functional correlates of low back pain in the elderly: the Iowa 65+ Rural Health Study. *J Am Geriatr Soc*, **33**, 23–8.

Leveille SG, Wee CC, and Iezzoni LI (1995). Trends in obesity and arthritis among baby boomers and their predecessors, 1971–2002. *Am J Public Health*, **95**, 1607–13.

Mobily PR, Herr KA, Clark MK, *et al.* (1994). An epidemiologic analysis of pain in the elderly. *J Aging Health*, **6**, 139–54.

O'Reilly SC, Muir KR, and Doherty M (1998). Knee pain and disability in the Nottingham community: association with poor health status and psychological distress. *Br J Rheumatol*, **37**, 870–3.

Papageorgiou AC, Croft PR, Ferry S, *et al.* (1995). Estimating the prevalence of low back pain in the general population. Evidence from the South Manchester Back Pain Survey. *Spine*, **20**, 1889–94.

Picavet HS and Schouten JS (2003). Musculoskeletal pain in the Netherlands: prevalences, consequences and risk groups, the DMC(3)-study. *Pain*, **102**, 167–78.

Saastamoinen P, Leino-Arjas P, Laaksonen M, *et al.* (2005). Socioeconomic differences in the prevalence of acute, chronic and disabling chronic pain among ageing employees. *Pain*, **114**, 364–71.

Scudds RJ and Østbye T (2001). Pain and pain-related interference with function in older Canadians: the Canadian study of health and aging. *Disabil Rehabil*, **23**, 654–64.

Thomas E, Peat G, Harris L, *et al.* (2004). The prevalence of pain and pain interference in a general population of older adults: cross-sectional findings from the North Staffordshire Osteoarthritis Project (NorStOP). *Pain*, **110**, 361–8.

Chapter 2

Assessment of pain, mood, and quality of life

S. José Closs

Key points

- Patient, proactive assessment of pain should be undertaken with older people, since many are reluctant to report it.
- For the majority, self report is the most accurate and reliable method of assessing pain, using simple pain intensity scales.
- For those who are unable to communicate their pain, a range of behavioural indicators may aid the identification of the presence of pain.
- Interactions between pain, depression, and anxiety make it essential to assess and treat (where appropriate) all three.

2.1 Introduction

Persistent pain is common in later life and, for many, is inextricably linked with negative mood states and a reduced quality of life. The 2001 UK National Census (National Statistics Online) indicated that pain or discomfort was reported by about half of over 65-year-olds, and 56% of men and 65% of women aged 75+ years. About 10–15% of those over 65 have depression, while about 5% have dementia (National Service Framework for Older People 2001). The prevalence of dementia rises to 62% in UK care homes (Matthews & Dening, 2002). Evidently pain is very common in older people and there is likely to be overlap between those in pain and those who have depression and/or dementia. There are complex interactions between pain, mood, and quality of life, and assessment of each of these may be necessary for many patients. Clinical assessments need to be brief and simple to use in practice, particularly those which need to be undertaken frequently and regularly.

Older people tend to be more reluctant to complain of pain and may have physical and mental changes which impede their ability to report pain. This should not lead to the assumption that their pain (or mood changes) are not significant. Although there is considerable research available which has investigated changes in pain perception with ageing, a review of this indicated that there was no convincing evidence that pain thresholds, tolerance, or ability to discriminate between pains are different for older people (Harkins, 2002). The American Geriatrics Society guidelines for the management of pain in older people reiterated that the most accurate and reliable evidence of the presence of pain and its intensity is the sufferer's report, as with any other age group (American Geriatrics Society Panel on Persistent Pain in Older Persons, 2002). Approaches to the assessment of pain (and also mood and quality of life) therefore can be fundamentally similar to those used with younger people, but need to take age-related attitudes and changes in health into consideration.

2.2 Assessing pain in older people—the need to be pro-active

Older people need to be asked proactively about their pain—many do not complain, for a variety of reasons. The attitudes and beliefs of older people may generate barriers to good pain control, usually through a reluctance to report pain. Older people are frequently stoic, believing that putting up with pain is the right and proper thing to do. Many have great faith in health-care professionals, and if they have consulted them once about their pain will then assume that everything possible is already being done, and will not report subsequent pain. Their religion may stop them from complaining if they feel that they are being punished for earlier sins. The meaning of their pain may also influence reporting, since admitting pain may be tantamount to acknowledging the presence of serious illness or impending death—denial may be their preferred coping strategy. They may also be afraid that if they report their pain, it might elicit unpleasant investigations or treatments.

Finally, they may not want to take analgesic drugs, due to unfounded fear of side effects or addiction. There is an important issue of education here, especially if analgesics are being avoided due to misconceptions about their effects.

It is not only attitudes and beliefs, but also health, i.e. physical and mental changes associated with ageing, which may impede pain assesment. Physical degeneration in sight, speech, or hearing, and cognitive

Box 2.1 The history

Should aim to identify and treat the underlying cause/s of pain (acute and/or chronic) and involve:

- Physical examination
- Diagnostic tests
- Psychological function
- Social situation and support
- Cognitive function.

impairment may all make understanding what is happening during an assessment difficult or impossible, and even if they are able to understand, they may not be able to express themselves adequately in order to communicate the presence of pain. Nevertheless, a thorough initial history (Box 2.1) should endeavour to elicit information from the patient using sight/hearing aids etc. where possible and from formal and informal carers where difficulties arise.

Subsequent regular assessments might use a 3-stage approach, first a general enquiry; second the use of pain intensity assessment instruments and third the use of behavioural pain scales where necessary.

2.3 Assessment through self-report of pain

It is important to set the scene for pain assessment carefully with each patient. Specific questions such as 'Do you have any pain or discomfort?' and 'Can you show me where it hurts?' are more likely to elicit a meaningful response than general questions such as 'Would you like something for the pain?'. The latter invites a polite 'No, thank you' type of response, whereas the former provides information about the pain itself. Using synonyms such as aching and soreness may be useful, since many would not use the word 'pain'. Asking in the present tense is often important where recall is poor, as is allowing time for patients to understand what they are being asked and to formulate their response. Patience is very important with this vulnerable group.

The location and intensity of pain are the simplest and probably the most useful aspects of pain to assess. Most patients are able to indicate location verbally or by pointing; and body charts may also be used with those who are able to use them. Simple pain intensity scales may be used in clinical situations where detailed approaches are neither feasible nor necessary. The two most appropriate scales for use with this population are the Numeric Rating Scale (NRS), (Figure 2.1) and the Verbal Rating Scale (VRS), (Figure 2.2), (American Geriatrics Society Panel on Persistent Pain in Older Persons, 2002;

Figure 2.1 Example of numeric rating scale (NRS) for pain intensity

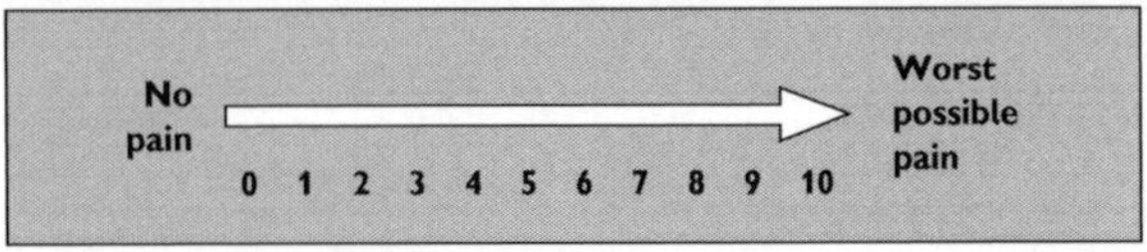

Figure 2.2 Example of verbal rating scale (VRS) for pain intensity

'Which of these best describes your pain right now?'

None	**Mild**	**Moderate**	**Severe**	**Excruciating**

Closs *et al.* 2004). The NRS involves a verbal enquiry as to how bad pain is on a scale of 1–10, where zero is no pain and ten is the worst pain possible, while a simple 5-point VRS would involve asking whether they would describe themselves as having (for example) no pain, mild, moderate, severe, or excruciating pain.

These scales may best be presented to patients in large print, for example on an A4 laminated sheet, allowing them to read and indicate their response. It may be helpful for the assessor to read out what is on the sheet at the same time.

Visual analogue scales (VAS) are widely used, typically presenting a simple 10 cm horizontal line, with an anchor statement at each end, such as 'no pain at all' at one end and 'worst pain imaginable' at the other. These are not particularly suitable for use with older people. Conceptually many older people find VAS difficult to grasp, and impaired dexterity may also make marking the line difficult.

2.4 Pain assessment through behavioural indicators of pain

For those with mild or moderate cognitive impairment, it is usually possible to self-report pain using simple, specific questions and simple pain intensity scales, as described above. For those with severe impairment, behavioural cues appear to be the only indicators from which the presence of pain may realistically be inferred. Over the past 5–10 years there has been an upsurge of interest in the development of instruments to assess pain in cognitively-impaired older people, allowing the publication of three reviews over the past year (Stolee *et al.* 2005; Herr *et al.* 2006; Zwakhalen *et al.* 2006).

Box 2.2 Observable indicators of the potential presence of pain

- Physiological cues—e.g. loss of appetite, flushing/blanching and perspiration.
- Verbalization—e.g. confused, aggressive or offensive speech.
- Vocalization—e.g. crying, groaning, screaming.
- Facial expression—e.g. wincing, rapid blinking, grimacing and other sad, distressed or distorted expressions.
- Body movements—e.g. rubbing of affected area, tension and guarding, altered gait, hand-wringing, repetitive movements, fidgeting and being generally unsettled.
- Mood changes—e.g. becoming easily upset; irritable, weepy, withdrawn, or confused.
- General behavioural changes—e.g. being quieter than usual, socially withdrawn, sleeping more frequently and at different times from usual, change of usual routines, and tendency to wander.

These instruments vary greatly, but tend to include seven main types of indicator, Box 2.2, (Hadjistavropoulos *et al.* 1999; Kovach *et al.* 2001; Cohen-Mansfield & Creedon, 2002).

Some instruments are fairly brief and simple, and might be appropriate for use in clinical practice, for example the Checklist of Nonverbal Pain Indicators (Feldt, 2000). Others are much longer and more comprehensive, such as the PACSLAC (Fuchs-Lacelle & Hadjistavropoulos, 2004) which lists 60+ items. The latter has better validity (to date) and is a promising research instrument but is too cumbersome for use in clinical practice. As yet there is no single instrument which has been shown to have psychometric properties sufficient for it to be recommended for clinical use.

Familiarity with the patient/client is very helpful when trying to understand the significance of individual behaviours. These behaviours vary enormously between individuals, occurring in different combinations and frequencies. What indicates pain in one person may indicate itching, fear, the need to go to the toilet etc. in another. The correct interpretation of behaviours depends to a great extent on familiarity with individuals. Family members may be well aware that a particular behaviour, such as pacing up and down, means that pain has worsened. Good communications between family/friends and health-care professionals should help in the interpretation of behavioural cues which may indicate the presence of pain.

2.5 Assessment of mood and quality of life in older people

Pain is associated with functional limitations, fatigue, sleeping problems, depressed mood, and quality of life in those aged over 75 (Jakobsson *et al.* 2003). There are complex interactions between these factors in older people. Many older people in persistent pain are both depressed and anxious; sleep deprivation can lead to anxiety; depression can be both the cause and the result of sleep disturbances; and depression and anxiety may exacerbate the pain experience. Treating one or more of these symptoms can produce improvements in others; for example, the treatment of depression in older adults with arthritis has been shown to improve not only depressive symptoms but also their pain, functional status, general health status, and overall quality of life (Lin *et al.* 2003). The assessment of these symptoms is therefore essential for many older people.

2.5.1 Depression and anxiety

In the UK, clinicians have tended to assess symptoms of depression and anxiety in older people using the instruments listed in Box 2.3.

Box 2.3 Instruments for assessment of depression and anxiety

- The **Beck Depression Inventory** (BDI) (Beck *et al.* 1961). This has 21 items whereby patients indicate which of four clustered statements describes their experience.
- The widely used **Hospital Anxiety and Depression scale** (HAD) (Zigmond & Snaith, 1983). This has 14 items which screen for both depression and anxiety, and was designed for use in a clinical setting.
- The **Spielberger StateTrait Anxiety Inventory** (STAI, Spielberger *et al.* 1983), which has a 20-item list of statements describing anxiety symptoms to be rated on four-point scales.
- The **Pain Anxiety Symptoms Scale** (PASS, McCracken *et al.* 1992), which includes 40 items which measure avoidance.

It is not clear from the literature which of these is most appropriate for use with older people in pain, but generally simpler scales such as the Hospital Anxiety and Depression Scale (HAD) are more suited for use with older people in clinical situations.

When the older person has difficulty in communicating, self-report scales are of questionable use. The selection of assessment scales depends on their purpose, and will vary according to the level of detail required and the nature of the population to be assessed. For some groups, such as nursing home residents with severe cognitive impairment, this presents considerable difficulties, and assessment may not always be possible. One scale designed for use with this group is the Affect Rating Scale (Lawton, 1994), which assesses outward signs of positive emotion (pleasure, interest, and contentment) and negative emotion (anger, anxiety, and depression).

2.5.2 Health-related quality of life

A review of the measurement properties of 15 quality of life instruments (Haywood *et al.* 2005) showed the best reliability, validity and responsiveness for the SF-36 (Ware 1997), EQ-5D (The EuroQol Group, 1990) and the NHP (Hunt *et al.* 1980). The most succinct of these was the EQ-5D, making it probably the most appropriate for use by clinicians, although the SF-36 was recommended for a more detailed health assessment. For older people who have difficulty communicating due to dementia or other problems, the 20-item Pleasant Events Schedule-AD (Logsdon & Teri, 1997) may be used to measure the person's participation in enjoyable activity, taking into account the frequency and apparent enjoyment of activities.

2.6 Conclusion

About half of the population of older people is likely to experience chronic pain. It is therefore important that clinicians assess and treat the cause and symptoms of pain wherever possible. From the brief overview presented in this chapter, the key issues to bear in mind when assessing the older person in pain are shown in Box 2.4.

Box 2.4 Assessing the older person in pain

1. Be proactive and patient. Many older people are reluctant to report their pain, and need time to understand and respond to assessment procedures. Introductory questions about pain should focus on specifics and use culturally appropriate language, including synonyms.
2. For those with more complex problems, a full history of their pain and related issues may be needed; for others simple location and intensity measures may suffice.
3. Self-report of pain is the most accurate and reliable approach to the assessment of pain. Simple pain intensity scales such as the NRS and VRS are particularly appropriate for older people.
4. For those who are unable to self-report due to cognitive impairment or other communication difficulties, behavioural indicators may be used. These may vary between individuals. Carers who are familiar with patients may be able to help in the interpretation of single or multiple behaviours.
5. Assessments of mood and quality of life may be important elements in the management of pain, with the enhanced treatment of one or more symptoms improving a range of others.

References

American Geriatrics Society Panel on Persistent Pain in Older Persons (2002). Clinical guideline: the management of persistent pain in older persons. *Journal of the American Geriatrics Society*, **50**, S205–S24.

Beck AT, Ward CH, Mendelson M, Mock J, and Erbaugh J (1961). An inventory for measuring depression. *Archives of General Psychiatry*, **4**, 561–71.

Closs SJ, Barr B, Briggs M, Cash K and Seers K (2004). A comparison of five pain assessment scales for nursing home residents with varying degrees of cognitive impairment. *Journal of Pain and Symptom Management*, **27**(3), 196–205.

Cohen-Mansfield J and Creedon M (2002). Nursing staff members' perceptions of pain indicators in persons with severe dementia. *Clinical Journal of Pain*, **18**(1), 64–73.

Department of Health (2001). *National Service Framework for Older People*. DoH, London.

The EuroQol Group (1990). EuroQol: A new facility for the measurement of health-related quality of life. *Health Policy*, **16**, 199–208.

Feldt KS (2000). Checklist of nonverbal pain indicators. *Pain Management Nursing*, **1**(1), 13–21.

Fuchs-Lacelle S and Hadjistavropoulos T (2004). Development and preliminary validation of the pain assessment checklist for seniors with limited ability to communicate (PACSLAC). *Pain Management Nursing*, **5**(1), 37–49.

Hadjistavropoulos T, LaChapelle DL, MacLeod FK, Snider B, and Craig K (1999). Measuring movement-exacerbated pain in cognitively impaired frail elders. *Clinical Journal of Pain*, **16**, 54–63.

Harkins S (2002). What is unique about the older adult's pain experience? In Weiner DK, Herr K, Rudy TE (eds). *Persistent Pain in Older Adults*. Springer Publishing Company, New York, pp.4–17.

Haywood KL, Garratt AM, and Fitzpatrick R (2005). Quality of life in older people: a structured review of generic self-assessed health instruments. *Quality of Life Research*, **14**, 1651–68.

Herr K, Bjoro K, and Decker S (2006). Tools for the assessment of pain in nonverbal older adults with dementia: a state-of-the-science review. *Journal of Pain and Symptom Management*, **31**(2), 170–92.

Hunt SM, McKenna SP, McEwen J, Backett EM, Williams J, and Papp E (1980). A quantitative approach to perceived health status: a validation study. *Journal of Epidemiology and Community Health*, **34**, 281–6.

Jakobsson U, Klevsgård R, Westergren A, and Hallberg IR (2003). Old people in pain: a comparative study. *Journal of Pain and Symptom Management*, **26**(1), 625–36.

Kovach CR, Noonan PE, Griffie J, Muchka S, and Weissman DE (2001). Use of the assessment of discomfort in dementia protocol. *Applied Nursing Research*, **14** (4), 193–200.

Lawton MP (1994). Quality of life in Alzheimer disease. *Alzheimer Disease and Associated Disorders*, **8** (Suppl 3), 138–50.

Lin EHB, Katon W, Von Korff M, Tang L, Williams JW. Jr, Kroenke K, *et al.* (2003). Effect of improving depression care on pain and functional outcomes among older adults with arthritis: a randomized controlled trial. *JAMA*, **290**(18), 2428–34.

Logsdon RG and Teri L (1997). The Pleasant Events Schedule-AD: psychometric properties and relationship to depression in Alzheimer's disease patients. *The Gerontologist*, **37**, 40–5.

Matthews FE and Dening T (2002). Prevalence of dementia in institutional care. *The Lancet*, **360**, 225–6.

McCracken LM, Zayfert C, and Gross RT (1992). The Pain Anxiety Symptoms Scale: development and validation of a scale to measure fear of pain. *Pain*, **50**, 67–73.

National Statistics Online. Self-reported health problems: by gender and age, 1996–7: Social Trends Dataset. www.statistics.gov.uk/statBase/xsdataset.asp?More=Y&vlnk=670&All=Y&B2.x=86&B2.y=13 (accessed 13/02/2007).

Spielberger CD, Gorsuch RL, Lushene R, Vagg PR, and Jacobs AG (1983). *Manual for the State-Trait Anxiety Inventory*. Consulting Psychologists Press, Palo Alto.

Stolee P, Hillier LM, Esbaugh J, Bol N, McKellar L, and Gauthier N (2005). Instruments for the assessment of pain in older persons with cognitive impairment. *Journal of the American Geriatrics Society*, **53**, 319–26.

Ware JE (1997). *SF-36 Health Survey. Manual and Interpretation Guide*. The Health Institute, New England Medical Centre, 2nd edn, Nimrod Press, Boston MA.

Zigmond AS and Snaith RP (1983). The hospital anxiety and depression scale. *Acta Psychiatrica Scandinavica*, **67**(6), 361–70.

Zwakhalen SMG, Hamers JPH, Abu-Saad HH, and Berger MPF (2006). Pain in elderly people with severe dementia: a systematic review of behavioural pain assessment tools. *BMC Geriatrics*, **6**(3), 15pp. Available at: www.biomedcentral.com/1471-2318/6/3.

20

Chapter 3

Pain in patients with cognitive impairment

Duncan Forsyth

Key points

- Pain is inadequately recognized and treated, especially in those with severe cognitive impairment.
- Poorly treated pain is associated with increased disability, depression, behavioural problems (inappropriate prescription of neuroleptics), and worsening cognitive function.
- Barriers to assessment of pain include: declining verbal communication skills with worsening dementia; most pain assessment scales rely upon verbal skills; and the misconception that pain is less severe in those with cognitive impairment.
- Better pain assessment should lead to better pain treatment and fewer risks associated with unrelieved pain.
- Correct detection, diagnosis and treatment requires appropriate training and properly validated and reliable assessment tools.
- A multifaceted approach using a combination of self-reported measures, surrogate pain reporting by family or carers, direct observation of potential pain indicators, monitoring for changes in usual activity and behaviour, and ruling pain out as a possible cause of behaviours through non-drug and analgesic trials, measures of functional impairment/change along with physiological or behavioural measures should improve the accuracy of pain assessment and improve the subsequent management of pain in this vulnerable group of older people.

3.1 Introduction

The fastest growing proportion of the population are those over 80 and it is this age group that are most likely to suffer and where dementia is most prevalent (Bernabei *et al.* 1998; Ferrell, 1995). So, the number of individuals with dementia who will suffer painful conditions will also rise. The verbalization of pain can be difficult for those who have cognitive impairment and may lead to under-treatment and under/mis-diagnosis. Unrelieved pain can have several adverse effects for the individual (Box 3.2), which may lead to inappropriate management, e.g. disruptive behaviour may be inappropriately treated by sedation rather than by assessment of and alleviation of the pain (Box 3.1). Failure to manage pain adequately in such individuals can also result in increased complaints and litigation by their family members (advocates). Thus, it is important that we understand how those with dementia perceive pain, that we recognize their pain and treat it.

Box 3.1 Case study A

An 80yr old male with a 4 year history of progressive cognitive decline was sent from his residential home to the medical assessment unit of his local hospital because of disturbed behaviour over the last 4 days. The care home reported that they would be happy to have him back once his aggression had resolved. His MMSE was unscoreable on admission as he would not answer any questions but was instead verbally abusive to the staff stating that he did not see the point of their f***ing questions. Urgent review by a consultant geriatrician was requested to agree that the patient should be sedated as he was also hitting the nursing staff in the medical assessment unit. When the consultant asked the patient about his behaviour he said "They keep f***ing hurting me, so I f***ing hit them". It transpired that he had fallen in the care home one week earlier and his behaviour had changed after that. X-ray revealed suspected humeral fracture and allowed adequate analgesia, careful handling and treatment. The next day he recognised the consultant and thanked him for sorting out his pain!

Box 3.2 Consequences of unrelieved pain

Acute

- Increased risk of complications:
  - Delirium
  - Deep vein thrombosis
  - Nausea and vomiting
  - Respiratory infections
- Increased mortality

Acute and chronic

- Behavioural changes
- Depression
- Psychosocial effects:
  - Isolation
  - Impaired mobility
  - Disrupted sleep
  - Changes in social roles and relationships
- Increased length of hospital stay
- Increased risk of institutionalization
- Decrease in successful rehabilitation
- Litigation

Box 3.3 Case study B

An 82-year-old male, with a 2-year history of progressive cognitive decline (MMSE 14/30) was admitted to hospital with a one-week history of worsening confusion and declining mobility such that his wife was no longer able to manage caring for him at home. The patient's sole complaint was of pain in the left knee. Physical and radiological examination of the knee were both normal. He was febrile with a raised white cell count and CRP. Serum urate and rheumatoid factor were normal. A routine chest X-ray revealed right middle lobe pneumonia. His pain disappeared with resolution of his pneumonia.

A thorough systematic assessment is required in cognitively impaired older people to reveal covert pathology and to investigate and remedy symptoms such as pain. The given history may not be accurate or may be absent, which can mislead the clinician (Boxes 3.3 and 3.4). Awareness of barriers that interfere with effective assessment and management of pain is important in developing a plan of care. The most obvious barrier is the inability of the person with severe dementia to communicate the presence of pain, at least in a manner that is easily understood, and to assist in the differentiation of pain aetiologies. This necessitates alternative approaches to assessment in this population, which are discussed below.

Box 3.4 Case study C

A 91-year-old female suffered a fractured right neck of femur three months previously. She had made good functional recovery and was discharged to her sheltered housing complex one month after surgery. Subsequently her daughters felt that she was managing badly at home and so one month later they moved her in to a residential home. Following this move mobility steadily declined and for the three days prior to being referred to hospital she was bedfast. Admission was finally precipitated because of a painful swollen left leg. MMSE on admission was zero (this was on a background of a six-year history of cognitive decline). A left DVT was diagnosed and she was started on anticoagulants. It was also noted that her left leg was obviously painful when moved despite her denying pain—she grimaced and gripped the sheets.

Some thought was needed!

- The DVT was the end result of failing mobility, so why was it failing?
- Also DVTs are not usually so painful. So was anything else wrong?
- She has fallen once before, could she have fallen again—she is so cognitively impaired that she would not remember or inform anyone.

The left leg was X-rayed. A left fractured neck of femur was confirmed.

3.2 Pain experience

Pain is an unpleasant sensory and emotional experience associated with actual or potential tissue damage or described in terms of such damage (Merskey & Bogduk, 1994). The experience of pain is, however, inherently subjective and will be modulated by a variety of factors, which include: mood state; perception of control; expectations; social conditioning; cultural conditioning and cognition (Figure 3.1). In a cognitively impaired individual both the experience and expression of pain may be altered. This poses difficulties in assessing pain and leads to persistent pain being under-reported, under-detected, and under-treated in the community as well as in institutions (Horgas & Tsai, 1998; Morrison & Siu, 2000). Selecting accurate and useful assessment instruments for use in those with cognitive impairment is a major problem. A recent review of 30 instruments for assessing pain in cognitively impaired older people found that none proved both reliable and valid and that for most reliability and validity data were basic or non-existent (Stolee *et al.* 2005). Thus, there is clearly a need for more rigorous development and testing of pain assessment instruments in cognitively impaired older people.

Figure 3.1 Triangle of pain characteristics

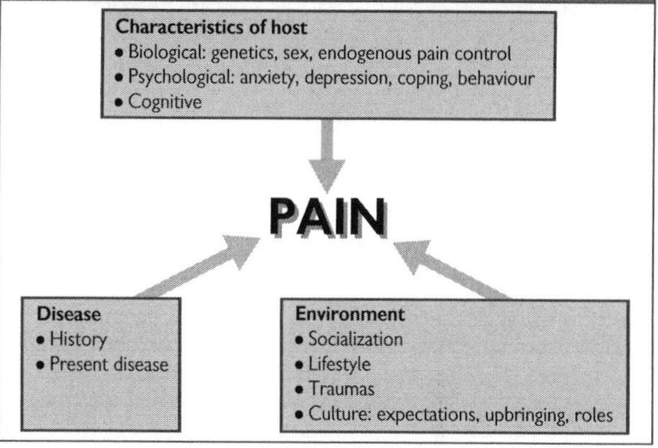

3.2.1 Language and pain

As language is a domain affected early in dementia, the individual's ability to communicate may be affected by their dementia, thereby impairing expression of pain, resulting in a substantial barrier to the assessment and management of pain. Pain assessment is only likely to be more problematic as disease advances. Indeed a study of 871 nursing home residents found that pain complaints and reported pain intensity declined with increasing cognitive impairment (Parmalee, 1996). No wonder then that although 79% of cognitively impaired nursing home residents may have a pain causing diagnosis fewer than 40% received any analgesia (Feldt *et al.* 1998a).

Many of the standardized pain assessment tools that are available are primarily forms of self-report. The verbalization of pain can be difficult for patients who have cognitive impairment, not only may they have problems responding to assessment instruments that require abstract thinking—localizing pain or describing its temporal relationship—but they may even have problems saying whether or not they have pain. Studies of pain and analgesia in cognitively intact and impaired older people with hip fracture have shown that both groups experience the same amount of pain (one-third had severe or very severe pain) but cognitively intact patients receive triple the amount of analgesia in the first 48 hours following surgery (Bell, 1997).

3.2.2 Non-verbal cues

As dementia progresses and verbal skills decline then carers and nursing and medical staff must increasingly rely on non-verbal cues of physical and emotional pain (Box 3.5). Common behaviours associated with pain are shown in Table 3.1; however, some patients demonstrate little or no specific behaviour associated with severe pain. Use of facial expressions or various behaviours may be difficult in patients who have Parkinson's disease or who have cerebrovascular damage.

3.2.3 Physiologic response to pain

There is no convincing evidence that peripheral nociceptor responses or pain transmission are impaired in older people. With increasing severity of dementia there is a blunting of the physiological response to pain (heart rate, respiratory rate), increased facial expression, and impaired ability to report anxiety and pain when exposed to venepuncture (Porter *et al.* 1996). Dementia sufferers have also been shown to suffer less from post lumbar puncture headache (Blennow *et al.* 1993). So, one might conclude, that an autonomic response to pain, in someone with dementia, suggests severe pain and the absence of an autonomic response does not mean absence of pain. It would also seem that dementia sufferers are less able to prepare for and perceive pain.

3.2.4 Correlation of pain experience with neuropathological changes

Using the acute versus chronic pain questionnaire (ACPQ) (Scherder *et al.* 2002) Alzheimer's patients have been shown to report more acute than chronic pain compared to controls, Alzheimer's patients also appear to be slower and less reliable in reporting a painful stimulus (Gibson *et al.* 2001). These findings correlate with the neuropathology of Alzheimer's. The medial pain system (hypothalamus, septohippocampal region, and amygdala) plays a significant role in the affective response to pain and is affected in Alzheimer's. Chronic pain is relayed to these limbic areas via the paleospinothalamic tract, whilst acute pain is relayed via the neospinothalamic tract to the somatic sensory cortex (lateral pain system). The lateral pain system is relatively well preserved in Alzheimer's. So Alzheimer's sufferers may perceive pain but have difficulty understanding and responding to it. Vascular dementia may lead to different patterns of pain interpretation dependent upon the site of vascular damage, e.g. thalamic infarction is associated with deafferentation pain; somatosensory cortical infarction may so impair the response to noxious stimuli that this leads to a reduction in chronic pain; and frontal infarction may affect the emotional response to pain.

Box 3.5 Non verbal cues in the expression of pain

- Agitation or irritability
- Repetitive verbalization/shouting
- Aggression
- Fluctuating cognition
- Falls/withdrawal
- Decreasing functional ability
- Sweating
- Tachycardia/raised blood pressure

Table 3.1 Common pain behaviours in cognitively impaired elderly persons

Facial expressions • Slight frown; sad, frightened face • Grimacing, wrinkled forehead, closed or tightened eyes • Any distorted expression • Rapid blinking	**Verbalizations** • Sighing, moaning, groaning • Grunting, chanting, calling out • Noisy breathing • Asking for help • Verbally abusive
Body movements • Rigid, tense body posture, guarding • Fidgeting • Repetitive rubbing of an area (perhaps indicating where pain is located) • Increased pacing, rocking • Restricted movement • Gait or mobility changes	**Changes in interpersonal interactions** • Aggressive, combative, resisting care • Decreased social interactions • Socially inappropriate, disruptive • Withdrawn
Changes in activity patterns or routines • Refusing food, appetite change • Increase in rest periods • Sleep, rest pattern changes • Sudden cessation of common routines • Increased wandering	**Mental status changes** • Crying or tears • Increased confusion • Irritability **Other restless or irritated behaviour** • Pulling at tubes

Table 3.1 is reproduced in modified form with permission from the American Geriatrics Society (2002). The Management of Persistant Pain in older persons. *Journal of the American Geriatrics Society*. Vol. **5**: 205–24. www.americangeriatrics.org

3.3 Age, cognition, and pain

3.3.1 Prevalence

Between 49% and 83% of community dwelling older people experience some form of pain of whom 10–15% suffer significant pain and up to 33% report daily persistent pain (Brochet *et al.* 1998). Similar rates are found in those with and without cognitive impairment (Mantyselka *et al.* 2004). Pain is also common in nursing home residents with an estimated 45–80% having substantial pain that is under-treated (Bernabei *et al.* 1998; Ferrell, 1995). One would anticipate that older people would experience more pain than their younger counterparts, as they suffer more physical illness and disability, yet older people report less pain than their younger counterparts and take/are prescribed fewer analgesics; those who are cognitively intact take more analgesics than those who are cognitively impaired (Sengstaken, 1993). See Chapter 1 for further discussion on epidemiology.

3.3.2 Prescribing of analgesia

Cognitively impaired nursing home residents are prescribed and administered significantly less analgesic medication, both in number and dosage, than their cognitively intact counterparts, even when they exhibit more behavioural indicators of pain, yet there is no evidence that cognitively impaired individuals have less pain or fewer painful conditions than cognitively intact individuals (Bell 1997; Feldt *et al.* 1998b; Horgas & Tsai 1998; Morrison & Siu, 2000). When the presence of diagnosed painful conditions was held constant, more disoriented and withdrawn patients were prescribed significantly less analgesia by physicians and administered less analgesia by nursing staff (Horgas & Tsai 1998). Even if pain experience is qualitatively different in dementia sufferers this is no excuse for neglect. Chronic unrelieved pain may have profound psychosocial effects such as isolation, impaired mobility, disrupted sleep, changes in social roles and relationships, and depression (See Box 3.2).

Despite the prevalence and consequences of pain amongst older people, health-care professionals remain ineffective at both its assessment (Hall-Lord, 1998; Weiner *et al.* 1999a) and its treatment (Bernabei, 1998; Morrison & Siu, 2000), especially in those who are unable to communicate their discomfort. Under-detection of pain in older people may be the result of several factors (Box 3.6), however the hypothesis that pain experience or perception diminish with ageing is unproven.

Box 3.6 Commonest reasons for the under-detection of pain in older people

- Reporting habits of older people
- Acceptance of reports by staff
- Ability of carers to identify pain (including inadequate training in pain management)
- Inappropriateness of existing pain measures
- Reluctance to prescribe for frail older people

3.4 Pain assessment scales

3.4.1 Sensory-discriminative assessment

Whilst evidence exists that older people with cognitive impairment can complete self-report pain scales (Chibnall & Tait, 2001; Closs *et al.* 2004; Taylor & Herr, 2003), a challenge remains in assessing pain in older people with more severe cognitive decline associated with a loss of language skills. Whilst self-report of pain is the gold standard for pain assessment, other approaches are necessary in this population, such as observational and surrogate reports. A precise and accurate method for interpreting the expression of pain in persons with cognitive impairment is not available. A variety of assessment scales exist for assessing pain (see Chapter 2 and Figure 3.2) the language and cognitive skills required vary from scale to scale.

3.4.2 Community dwelling elders with cognitive impairment

In a community-based study in Finland, Mantyselka *et al.* (2004), using multidimensional pain assessment, found that 85% with mild–moderate dementia could answer questions regarding pain compared to only 20% of those with severe dementia. Krulewitch (2000) evaluated the responses of community dwelling elders with cognitive impairment and their caregivers on three pain assessment measures. One-third of the cognitively impaired individuals were unable to complete any pain assessment tool; of those completing at least one assessment tool 87.5% reported some pain. For those able to complete an assessment there was 67% agreement between the assessment of the patient and the caregiver as to the level of pain. The Pain Intensity Scale was the tool most likely to be completed by both patients and caregivers.

3.4.3 Nursing home residents with cognitive impairment

Dementia is the single commonest reason for institutionalization with a prevalence in excess of 50% in nursing home residents. Pain prevalence studies in nursing home residents reveal rates varying

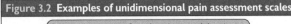

Figure 3.2 Examples of unidimensional pain assessment scales

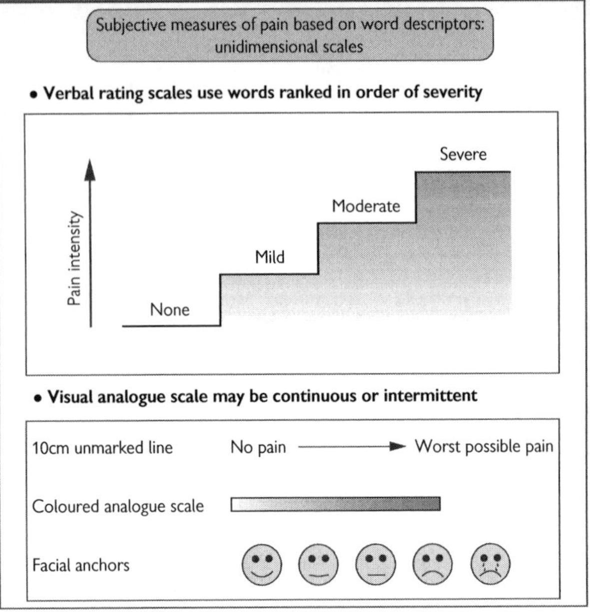

from 45–80%, mostly musculoskeletal. In a study evaluating pain in nursing home residents, 33% of the patients were excluded (primarily because they were comatose), most of the remainder had significant cognitive impairment; of the remainder 62% had pain complaints, 83% of whom could complete at least one unidimensional scale (Ferrell *et al.* 1995). Ferrell (1995) has also shown that 1 in 3 of 112 NH residents with mild–moderate dementia could complete all of five unidimensional scales. As the cognitive and language skills required to complete pain assessment tools increase then the ability of nursing home residents to complete these tools declines (Figure 3.3) (Ferrell, 1995; Ferrell *et al.* 1995). Manz (2000) found that patients with moderate to no cognitive impairment were able to complete one or more pain assessment tools; only 30% of those with severe cognitive impairment could complete at least one pain assessment tool. So it would seem that pain is common in cognitively impaired individuals and may be assessable using simple scales. However, Ferrell (1995) did question whether the dementia sufferers who completed a pain scale understood what they were doing and were able to give accurate responses.

Figure 3.3 Derived completion rates for 325 residents in a nursing home of pain assessment scales

Derived completion rates, for 325 residents in a nursing home, of pain assessment scales used by Ferrell *et al.* (1995) and a description of the skills required to complete each measure

Measure	Skills required to complete measure	Completion rate
Ferrell Pain Questionnaire for the Elderly	Unclear, as insufficient information provided	79%
McGill Pain Questionnaire	Recognition of words, written and spoken, ability to point	63%
McGill Present Pain Intensity Scale	Recognition of words, written and spoken, ability to point	51%
Memorial Pain card (modified Tursky Scale)	Recognition of words, written and spoken, ability to point	47%
Rand COOP Chart for Pain	Recognition of pictures or words written and spoken, ability to point	45%
Verbal analogue scale	Abstract thought required to translate pain experience into numbers, recall of past pain states, ability to answer verbally	37%
100mm visual analogue scale	Abstract thought to translate pain onto line, recall of past pain states, ability to use pencil	35%

3.4.4 **Hospitalized patients with severe cognitive impairment**

Sixty-one percent of 129 severely demented, hospitalised patients (mean age 83.7 years, 69% women) were able to comprehend at least one of three self-assessment tools—the verbal, horizontal visual, and faces pain scales. Comprehension rates were significantly better for the verbal and the faces pain scales. Observational rating of pain by nursing staff correlated at least moderately with self-assessment ($r = 0.25$–0.63). However, the observational rating scale underestimated pain severity compared with all three self-assessment scales (Pautex *et al.* 2006).

People with mild cognitive impairment are less likely to report pain to carers or nurses, but are able to describe their experience accurately when prompted. Those with cognitive impairment may be more likely to report pain to a carer using a pain assessment tool

Figure 3.3 is reproduced from *J. Pain Symptom Manage.* **10**, Ferrell, B.A., Ferrell, B.R., Rivera, L. Pain in cognitively impaired nursing home patients, pp. 591–8, © (1995), with permission from the US Cancer Pain Relief Committee and Elsevier.

rather than if they are simply asked 'Do you have any pain?'. Unidimensional scales may be easier to use, with one study showing that 73% of patients with cognitive impairment could use a verbal rating scale (ranging from 'slight pain' to 'pain as bad as it could be'). So, perhaps the emphasis need not necessarily be on the method of pain assessment, but that pain should be assessed by some method!

The processing of these sensory-discriminative aspects of pain occurs in the lateral pain system which is preserved in Alzheimer's dementia.

3.5 Motivational-affective assessment

3.5.1 In non-communicative individuals

Pain assessment in non-communicative individuals largely relies upon attention to behaviour (Box 3.7). These observational scales are based upon recognizing the behaviours identified in Table 3.1. Individuals with cognitive impairment present with a unique 'pain signature'. Whereas one person may become withdrawn and quiet, another may become agitated. Both of these behaviour patterns could indicate pain, but are difficult to reconcile with behavioural tools that attempt to score behaviours by pain intensity and that are narrow in the indicators included. The strengths and limitations of these nonverbal assessment tools have recently been reviewed (Herr *et al.* 2006) to guide the clinician in selecting a tool appropriate for the patient and setting. Use of these tools in minority older adults with dementia is limited.

Box 3.7 Observational pain assessment scales in non-communicative individuals

- DS-DAT (discomfort scale dementia Alzheimer's type)
- CNPI (checklist of nonverbal pain indicators)
- Assessment of discomfort in dementia
- Pain behaviour measure
- Proxy pain questionnaire
- Facial action coding system
- Pain assessment for dementing elderly
- Doloplus 2
- Behaviour checklist
- Facial grimace scale
- Elderly pain caring assessment
- Pain assessment checklist for seniors with severe dementia (PACSLAC)
- Nursing assistant-administered instrument to assess pain in demented individuals (NOPPAIN)
- Pain assessment in advanced dementia (PAINAD)

These measure frowning, grimacing, abnormal posture (latter may be abnormal due to extrapyramidal syndromes).

The processing of these motivational-affective aspects of pain occurs in the medial pain system, which is affected in Alzheimer's dementia. This can result in people with dementia having altered affective responses to pain, due to their inability to cognitively process the painful sensation in the context of prior pain experience, attitudes, knowledge, and beliefs. Reactions to painful sensations may therefore differ from the typical response expected from a cognitively intact older person. For example, constipation can cause great distress in the cognitively impaired older person and may lead to aggressive or agitated behaviours. As there is no evidence that those with dementia experience less pain, we should assume that any condition that is painful to a cognitively intact person would also be painful to those with advanced dementia who cannot express themselves. For example, pain should be considered as a possible explanation for a change in behaviour in an older person with advanced dementia (Table 3.1). Although subtle changes in usual patterns of behaviour or activity do not always mean that the patient is in pain, they should raise the suspicion and lead to a thorough evaluation for possible pain-causing problems.

As many severely demented patients are capable of reliably reporting their own pain, observational scales need only be relied upon in those individuals who can not verbally report pain.

3.5.2 **Interpretation of pain behaviour by different assessors**

Whilst observation of behaviours and activities that may indicate pain is fundamental to the assessment of those with advanced dementia who are unable to verbally report their pain experience, it can be difficult to recognize that certain behaviours may indicate pain if the health or social care provider is unfamiliar with how the person usually behaves. It has been conjectured that care home staff may improve in pain detection as they get to know residents. Therefore, it is imperative to improve health and social care professionals' knowledge and skills related to pain assessment and aggressive approaches to comprehensive pain assessment be adopted. Using rapid cycle quality improvement programme Baier *et al.* (2004) achieved a 41% reduction in residents' pain in 17 intervention nursing homes compared to a 19% reduction in all 95 nursing homes in Rhode Island. In the intervention group the assessment of pain rose from 4 to 44% and the use of pain assessment scales rose from 16 to 74%. When compared with patient self-reported pain ratings well-trained care-giver surrogates appear to rate an individual's pain accurately (Dirks, 1993; Weiner *et al.* 1999a); health-care surrogates (both physicians and nurses) tend to underestimate the severity of the patient's pain (Cohen-Mansfield & Lipson, 2002; Hall-Lord *et al.* 1998; Horgas & Dunn, 2001; Weiner *et al.* 1999); and family caregivers, although more adept at estimating the pain of others, tend to overestimate the intensity of pain (Cohen-Mansfield, 2002). So, although surrogate reporters are able to recognize the presence of pain they have difficulty accurately identifying the severity of pain from behavioural observation (Shega *et al.* 2004). Simply observing an individual at rest may not identify pain behaviours which may only occur during activities such as transferring, walking and repositioning (Feldt *et al.* 1998b; Hadjistavropolous *et al.* 2000; Weiner *et al.* 1996). So, care staff need to be trained to observe for pain behaviour and to understand that this may only be evident when the painful body part is used, e.g. a fractured pelvis may not hurt whilst lying still in bed but will hurt when turning over or being assisted to the toilet. However, even if we recognize that someone is in pain that does not necessarily mean that we are able to quantify how much pain they are in. In the verbally non-communicative individual with cognitive impairment the following algorithm provides a basis for assessing and managing pain-related behaviour (Figure 3.4).

Figure 3.4 Algorithm for assessing pain in verbally non-communicative older people (adapted from Weiner *et al.* 2002)

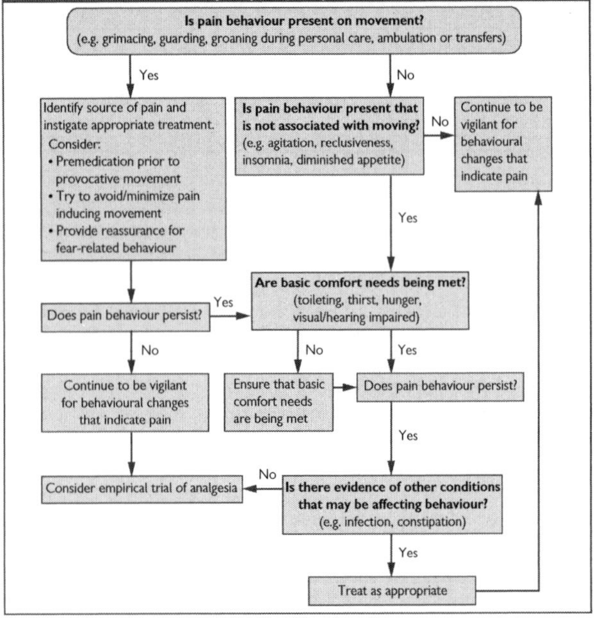

Figure 3.4 is reproduced from Weiner, D., Herr, K., Rudy, T. (eds) (2002). Persistent Pain in Older Adults: An Interdisciplinary Guide for Treatment. Springer Publishing Company, New york, with permission from Dr Weiner.

3.6 Quality of life

Adequate pain assessment forms the basis for optimal pain control, has major implications for quality of life (QoL) and quality of care of older people (Box 3.8). Unrelieved pain has been associated with altered immune function, impaired psychological function (e.g., depression, anxiety, fear), impaired physical function (e.g., impaired mobility and gait, delayed rehabilitation, falls), sleep disturbance, compromised cognitive function, and decreased socialization (AGS 2002; Brummel-Smith *et al.* 2002; Landi *et al.* 2005; Schuler *et al.* 2004; Weiner *et al.* 2002). These may all result in increased dependency as well as increased use of health-care resources, with resultant increased costs. In those with severe cognitive impairment it is all too easy to attribute these effects to their dementia, rather than to unrecognized and untreated painful conditions. For instance, demented patients with persistent pain are more likely to be treated with benzodiazepines and antipsychotics than their non-demented counterparts (Balfour & O'Rouke, 2003).

Box 3.8 Untreated pain may adversely affect pre-existing cognitive impairment and result in inappropriate management

Cognitive change
- Poor concentration

Psychological change
- Depression
- Anxiety
- Sleep disturbance

Behavioural change
- Restlessness
- Irritability
- Apathy
- Decreased socialisation
- Altered mobility (decreased or wandering)

This may result in increasing care needs due to:
- Increased depression
- Increased challenging behaviour
- Increased vocalization
- Slower rehabilitation
- Effects of polypharmacy

Box 3.9 Non-pharmacological measures to relieve pain behaviours

- Supportive verbal communication
- Music therapy
- Therapeutic massage
- Soothing/supportive touch
- Cold or heat therapy
- Physical exercise/movement

3.7 Analgesic trial

An empiric trial of analgesia may be warranted if pain behaviours persist after other possible causes are ruled out or treated. Choice of appropriate analgesic is challenging because it is difficult to determine the level of pain severity in persons with advanced dementia. Starting with paracetamol seems prudent (Kovach *et al.* 2002) whilst titration to stronger analgesics may be necessary before ruling out pain as the aetiology for behaviour or activity changes. If analgesic use results in decreased pain related behaviours, it seems reasonable to assume that pain was the likely cause and continue pharmacologic and/or nonpharmacologic interventions (Box 3.9) (Kovach *et al.* 2002). The increased susceptibility of cognitively impaired older people to adverse drug effects clearly necessitates very careful monitoring of any analgesic trial.

3.8 Recommendations and learning points

- Better pain assessment should lead to better pain treatment and fewer risks associated with unrelieved pain.
- Correct detection, diagnosis, and treatment requires appropriate training and properly validated and reliable assessment tools.
- A multifaceted approach using a combination of self-reported measures, family or carer input, measures of functional impairment/change, along with physiological or behavioural measures should improve the accuracy of pain assessment and improve the subsequent management of pain in this vulnerable group of older people.

In a communicative individual with cognitive impairment the following tips will assist in the assessment of pain:

- Frame questions in the here and now.
- Use concrete questions with yes/no responses.
- Repete the question.

* Use validating questions.
* Ensure communication aids (spectacles, hearing aids) are worn and functioning.
* Give adequate time for the individual to respond to questions.

References

American Geriatrics Society Panel on Persistent Pain in Older Persons (2002). Clinical practice guidelines: The management of persistent pain in older persons. *JAGS*, **50**, S205–24.

Baier RR, Gifford DR, Patry G, *et al.* (2004). Ameliorating pain in nursing homes: a collaborative quality improvement project. *JAGS*, **52**, 2138–40.

Balfour JE and O'Rourke N (2003). Older adults with Alzheimer disease, comorbid arthritis and prescription of psychotropic medications. *Pain Res Manag*, **8**, 198–204.

Bell ML (1997). Postoperative pain management for the cognitively impaired older adult. *Semin Perioper Nurs*, **6**, 37–41.

Bernabei R, Gambassi G, Lapane K, *et al.* (1998). Management of pain in elderly patients with cancer. The SAGE Study Group (Systematic Assessment of Geriatric drug use via Epidemiology). *JAMA*, **279**, 1877–82.

Blennow K, Wallin A, Hager O (1993). Low frequency of post-lumbar puncture headache in demented patients. *Acta Neurol Scand*, **88**, 221–3.

Brochet B, Michel P, Barberger-Gateau P, *et al.* (1998). Population-based study of pain in elderly people: a descriptive survey. *Age and Ageing*, **27**, 279–84.

Brummel-Smith K, London MR, Drew N, *et al.* (2002). Outcomes of pain in frail older adults with dementia. *JAGS*, **50**, 1847–51.

Chibnall J and Tait R (2001). Pain assessment in cognitively impaired and unimpaired older adults: A comparison of four scales. *Pain*, **92**, 173–86.

Closs SJ, Barr B, Briggs M, *et al.* (2004). A comparison of five pain assessment scales for nursing home residents with varying degrees of cognitive impairment. *J Pain Symptom Manage*, **27**, 196–204.

Cohen-Mansfield J (2002). Relatives' assessment of pain in cognitively impaired nursing home residents. *J Pain Symptom Manage*, **4**, 562–71.

Cohen-Mansfield J, and Lipson S (2002). Pain in cognitively impaired nursing home residents: How well are physicians diagnosing it? *JAGS*, **50**, 1039–44.

Dirks JF, Wunder J, Kingsman R, *et al.* (1993). A pain rating scale and pain behavior checklist for clinical use: Development, norms, and the consistency score. *Psychother Psychosomat*, **59**, 41–9.

Feldt KS, Ryden MB, Miles S. (1998b). Treatment of pain in cognitively impaired compared with cognitively intact older patients with hip fracture. *JAGS*, **46**, 1079–85.

Feldt KS, Warne MA, Ryden MB. (1998a). Examining pain in aggressive cognitively impaired older adults. *J Gerontol Nurs*, **24**, 14–22.

Ferrell BA (1995). Pain evaluation and management in the nursing home. *Ann Intern Med*, **123**, 681–7.

Ferrell BA, Ferrell BR, and Rivera L (1995). Pain in cognitively impaired nursing home patients. *J Pain Symptom Manage*, **10**, 591–8.

Gibson SJ, Voukelatos X, Ames D, *et al.* (2001). An examination of pain perception and cerebral event-related potentials following carbon dioxide laser stimulation in patients with Alzheimer's disease and age-matched control volunteers. *Pain Res Manag*, **6**, 126–32.

Hadjistravropolous T, LaChapelle D, MacLeod F, *et al.* (2000). Measuring movement-exacerbated pain in cognitively impaired frail elders. *Clin J Pain*, **16**, 54–63.

Hall-Lord ML, Larrson G, and Steen B (1998). Pain and distress among elderly intensive care unit patients: Comparison of patients' experiences and nurses' assessments. *Heart and Lung*, **27**, 123–32.

Herr K, Bjoro K, Decker S (2006). Tools for assessment of pain in nonverbal older adults with dementia: a state-of-the-science review. *J Pain Symptom Manage*, **31**, 170–92.

Horgas AL and Dunn K (2001). Pain in nursing home residents: Comparison of residents' self-report and nursing assistants' perceptions. *J Gerontol Nurs*, **27**, 44–53.

Horgas AL and Tsai PF (1998). Analgesic drug prescription and use in cognitively impaired nursing home residents. *Nurs Res*, **47**, 235–42.

Kovach C, Noonan P, Griffie J, *et al.* (2002).The assessment of discomfort in dementia protocol. *Pain Manag Nurs*, **3**, 16–27.

Krulewitch H, London M, Skakel V, *et al.* (2000). Assessment of pain in cognitively impaired older adults: a comparison of pain assessment tools and their use by non-professional caregivers. *JAGS*, **48**, 1607–11.

Landi F, Onder G, Cesari M, *et al.* (2005). Pain and its relation to depressive symptoms in frail older people living in the community: An observational study. *J Pain Symptom Manage*, **29**, 255–62.

Mantyselka P, Hartikainen S, Louhivuori-Laako K *et al.* (2004). Effects of dementia on perceived daily pain in home-dwelling elderly people: a population-based study. *Age & Ageing*, **33**, 496–9.

Manz B, Mosier R, Nusser-Gerlach M, *et al.* (2000). Pain assessment in the cognitively impaired and unimpaired elderly. *Pain Manag Nurs*, **1**, 106–15.

Merskey H, Bogduk N (eds.) (1994). *Classification of Chronic Pain, Second Edition.* IASP Task Force on Taxonomy. IASP Press, Seattle. pp. 209–14.

Morrison RS and Siu AL (2000). A comparison of pain and its treatment in advanced dementia and cognitively intact patients with hip fracture. *J Pain Symptom Manage*, **19**, 240–8.

Parmelee PA (1996). Pain in cognitively impaired older persons. *Clin Geriatr*, **12**, 473–87.

Pautex S, Michon A, Guedira M, *et al.* (2006). Pain in severe dementia: self-assessment or observational scales? *JAGS*, **54**, 1040–5.

Porter FL, Malhotra KM, Wolf CM, *et al.* (1996). Dementia and response to pain in the elderly. *Pain*, **68**, 413–21.

Scherder EJ, Smit R, Vuijk PJ, *et al.* (2002). The Acute versus Chronic Pain Questionnaire (ACPQ) and actual pain experience in older people. *Aging Ment Health*, 6, 304–12.

Schuler M, Njoo N, Hestermann M, *et al.* (2004). Acute and chronic pain in geriatrics: Clinical characteristics of pain and the influence of cognition. *Pain Med*, **5**, 253–62.

Sengstaken EA and King SA. (1993). The problems of pain and its detection among geriatric nursing home residents. *JAGS*, **41**, 541–4.

Shega JW, Hougham GW, Stocking CB, *et al.* (2004). Pain in community-dwelling persons with dementia: frequency, intensity, and congruence between patient and caregiver report. *J Pain Symptom Manage*, **28**, 585–92.

Stolee P, Hillier IM, Esbaugh J, *et al.* (2005) Instruments for the assessment of pain in older persons with cognitive impairment. *JAGS*, **53**, 319–26.

Snow AL, Weber JB, O'Malley KJ, *et al.* (2004). NOPPAIN: A nursing assistant-administered pain assessment instrument for use in dementia. *Dement Geriatr Cogn Disord*, **17**, 240–6.

Taylor LJ and Herr K (2003). Pain intensity assessment: a comparison of selected pain intensity scales for use in cognitively intact and cognitively impaired African-American older adults. *Pain Manag Nurs*, **4**, 87–95.

Weiner D, Pieper C, McConnell E, *et al.* (1996). Pain measurement in elders with chronic low back pain: traditional and alternative approaches. *Pain*, **67**, 461–7.

Weiner D, Peterson B, and Keefe F. (1999). Chronic pain-associated behaviours in the nursing home: resident versus caregiver perceptions. *Pain*, **80**, 577–88.

Weiner D, Herr K, and Rudy T (eds.) (2002). *Persistent pain in older adults: An interdisciplinary guide for treatment.* Springer Publishing Company, New York.

Chapter 4

Osteoporosis

Caitlyn Dowson

Key points

- Established osteoporosis (i.e. with fractures) is a common cause of acute and chronic pain in older people.
- These pains are multifactorial in origin and require careful assessment.
- Other painful underlying pathologies must be excluded.
- A wide variety of interventions exist to reduce pain in osteoporosis.
- These must be tailored to the needs of each older person.
- A multidisciplinary team is required.

4.1 Introduction

Osteoporosis is often described in books, but not by sufferers, as a painless condition or silent menace. It is a common chronic condition among older people that is 'characterized by low bone mass and micro-architectural deterioration of bone tissue, leading to enhanced bone fragility and a consequent increase in fracture risk' (World Health Organization, 1994). This is due to an imbalance in the remodelling process, with bone resorption exceeding bone formation. This tends to progress unnoticed for many years until a painful fracture occurs or deformity and disability develop. However, osteoporosis must not be accepted as an inevitable fact of later life. Effective interventions are available to reduce the risks for developing osteoporosis and fractures and it would be wrong to assume that age is a barrier to treatment.

4.2 Clinical features

4.2.1 Acute pain

Severe acute pain follows fractures that may occur spontaneously or follow relatively minor trauma. Low trauma fractures are generally defined as fractures occurring following a fall from standing or less.

Vertebral, hip, and wrist fractures are classically associated with osteoporosis but any bone may be affected. The degree of pain experienced following a vertebral fracture varies greatly among individuals from none at all to excruciating and incapacitating. Acute pain derives from the fractured vertebra, associated soft tissue damage, and the associated powerful reflex muscle spasm (Figure 4.1). The pain from the fractured vertebra will be well localized by the patient and will be tender to palpation. The painful muscle spasm may be more diffuse but is usually clearly evident on examination. Extruding bony fragments causing nerve root or spinal cord compression will produce referred pain and sphincter dysfunction according to the level involved. Pain referred to the ribs or abdomen is common. Erect posture, movement of the spine, inspiration and coughing may aggravate all of these pains. Patients may also find it unbearable to lie down.

Figure 4.1 Acute pain of vertebral fractures

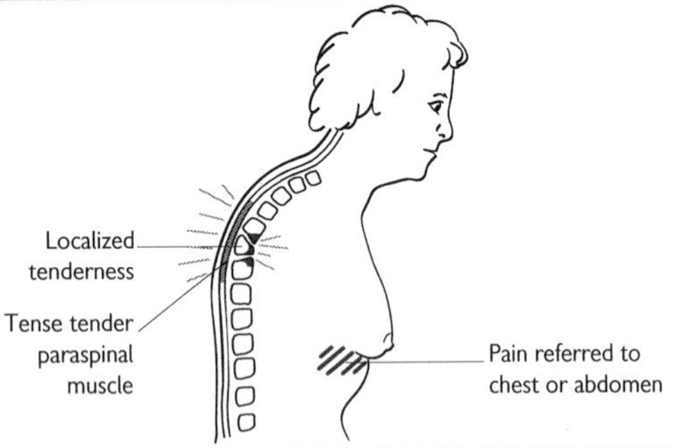

Hip fractures that occur following minimal trauma, such as a fall from standing, should arouse strong suspicion of osteoporosis or a more sinister underlying pathology. Older people, especially those already taking analgesia for other painful conditions, may not necessarily complain of the severe pain usually associated with traumatic hip fractures and may continue to bear weight following a fall.

Pain due to insufficiency fractures of the sacrum or pubic rami may not be well localized and the fractures sometimes missed on plain X-ray.

As the pain experienced following a fracture is so variable among older people, any trauma, however mild, requires careful assessment.

4.2.2 **Chronic pain**

Although the severe pain following a fracture usually settles within six to ten weeks many elderly patients are left with a variety of chronic pains. Pain persists beyond the expected healing time due to chronic muscle spasm, non-union, neuropathy, deformity or secondary osteoarthritis (Figure 4.2). The Dowager's hump is the classical deformity of osteoporosis. Kyphosis can occur following a single vertebral fracture, if the anterior aspect has collapsed entirely leaving a wedge-shaped vertebra, and becomes more marked with multiple fractures. Kyphotic patients experience chronic mechanical back pain due to ligament strain resulting from their abnormal posture and altered centre of gravity. Painful muscle spasm is common around the neck and shoulders as increased neck extension is required to look straight ahead. With severe kyphosis, the inferior ribs impinge painfully on the pelvis, the abdomen protrudes, and limited diaphragm movement causes shortness of breath and ultimately respiratory failure.

Figure 4.2 Chronic pain of established osteoporosis

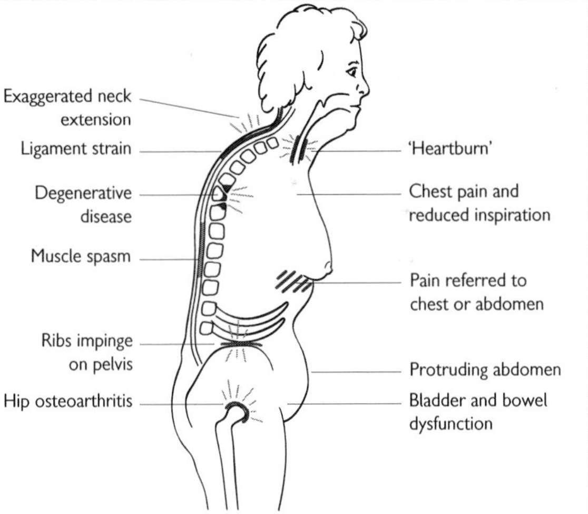

Painful secondary degenerative changes of the fractured and adjacent vertebrae and discs commonly develop. Associated facet joint involvement and nerve root impingement add to the cocktail of pain experienced by the older person with established osteoporosis.

Whilst kyphosis is generally well recognized, other less obvious deformities may contribute to chronic pain. A leg length discrepancy following a hip fracture will produce a pelvic tilt, scoliosis, and low back pain with or without nerve root irritation. Secondary osteoarthritis may develop in the fractured hip or in the opposite hip and knee if they are bearing more weight. Likewise, chronic shoulder pain develops due to reliance on walking aids and low back pain may be aggravated by long-term wheelchair use.

Established osteoporosis is associated with significant morbidity, mortality and reduced quality of life (Lips & Van Schoor, 2005). Very few regain their previous level of activity and independence. The resultant loss of confidence, social isolation and depression impact on older people's ability to manage their condition and in particular their pain.

4.2.3 **Underlying pathology**

Neither acute nor chronic musculoskeletal pain (nor low bone density) in older patients can be assumed to be due to osteoporosis until other significant pathology has been excluded.

Underlying metabolic bone disease, such as osteomalacia or hyperparathyroidism, may be contributing to the chronic musculoskeletal pain. Care home residents with severe vitamin D deficiency suffer widespread deep pain and tenderness, muscle weakness, and insufficiency fractures due to osteomalacia. Supplementation improves pain and muscle strength and reduces the risk for falls and fractures (Venning, 2005).

Severe unremitting pain and systemic upset suggest malignancy or infection until proven otherwise. Myeloma and metastases must be excluded. Similarly, not all kyphosis is due to osteoporotic vertebral collapse. Severe degenerative disc disease or ankylosing spondylitis may produce similar deformity, loss of height and a variety of acute and chronic pains.

4.3 Management

Dual energy X-ray absorptiometry (DEXA) is used to establish the diagnosis of osteoporosis. Plain X-ray, magnetic resonance imaging (MRI) and a range of blood tests may be required to exclude underlying causes. It is important to identify and minimise risks for osteoporosis, falls and fractures (Box 4.1).

Box 4.1 Risk factors for osteoporosis

- Low trauma fracture
- Low body mass index
- Parental history of osteoporosis
- Untreated premature menopause
- Prolonged immobility
- Medical condition associated with osteoporosis
- Medication—corticosteroids, anticonvulsants
- Smoking, alcohol abuse and poor calcium intake

Management of the older patient with osteoporosis also requires careful evaluation and treatment of the presenting pain. Due to the multifactorial nature of pain in osteoporosis, a multifaceted approach to relieve it is essential (Box 4.2).

Box 4.2 Multifaceted approach to pain management

- Surgery
- Analgesia
- Physical therapies
- Interventional radiology
- Psychological support

4.3.1 Surgery

General principles for the management of fractures apply, but may be more challenging to implement due to poor bone quality and other comorbidities. Hip fractures invariably require surgical intervention for pain relief and to regain mobility. The procedure performed depends on the site and severity of the fracture and the general health of the patient. Without surgical intervention, an older patient is very unlikely to become ambulant again. A multidisciplinary care package, tailored to the needs of the frail is essential to reduce the associated high morbidity and mortality (Morrison *et al.* 1998; Roche *et al.* 2005). Severe secondary osteoarthritis following fractures may become very painful and relieved only with joint replacement.

Spinal fusion is occasionally required to relieve severe pain from vertebral fractures but is hindered by the poor bone quality of adjacent vertebrae. Rib and pelvic fractures generally do not warrant surgical intervention but sufferers often still require the medical, physical and psychological support offered to patients with vertebral or hip fractures.

4.3.2 **Analgesia**

Analgesia must be initiated at an appropriate level and titrated in accordance with the severity of pain. A regular regimen should be recommended rather than waiting until the pain becomes severe.

Paracetamol may be all that is required but it is usually used in combination with other analgesic agents. Non-steroidal anti-inflammatory drugs are beneficial for bone pain following fracture and for subsequent osteoarthritis, but are often contraindicated in older patients. Steroid plus lignocaine joint injections may be beneficial if the osteoarthritic joint appears inflamed (and infection has been excluded).

Opiates, when used with care, provide powerful pain relief and improve outcomes for patients with osteoporotic fractures (Morrison *et al.* 2003). Associated drowsiness, poor balance and increased risks for further falls and fractures, are of particular concern in the older patient with osteoporosis. Constipation is another major problem, especially for patients with acute vertebral fractures (which may be associated with ileus), where straining at the toilet can be extremely painful and result in further vertebral fractures. A variety of laxatives will be required and should be commenced before constipation develops in this group of patients. The risk of opioid induced respiratory suppression is even greater in older patients with restricted painful respiration and a concoction of analgesic agents, muscle relaxants and sleeping tablets. Deep breathing exercises are required to reduce the risk for developing pneumonia.

Calcitonin (subcutaneous and possibly intranasal) has analgesic properties, in addition to its beneficial effects on bone density and fractures, and has been shown to reduce the duration and severity of acute pain if given within the first few weeks following vertebral fracture (Knopp *et al.* 2005). Intravenous pamidronate is also used for this purpose.

4.3.3 **Physical therapies**

The expert input of a physiotherapist with a special interest in managing older patients with osteoporotic fractures is required to optimize mobility, and to reduce both the acute and chronic pains described above (Malmros *et al.* 1998) (Box 4.3).

Whilst a brief period of bed rest may help to ease pain, early mobilization is preferable to reduce complications due to immobility, including further bone loss. Muscle spasm, whether acute or chronic, may be eased with massage, heat, cold, transcutaneous electronic nerve stimulation (TENS), acupuncture and specific exercises. Hydrotherapy may be beneficial during the recovery period, depending

Box 4.3 Physical therapies

- Physiotherapy
- Brief bed rest
- Early mobilization
- Massage
- Hot or cold compress
- Transcutaneous electronic nerve stimulation (TENS)
- Acupuncture
- Stretching and strengthening exercises
- Hydrotherapy
- Adjuvant analgesics and muscle relaxants

on the severity of the pain, degree of mobility and absence of contra-indications (Chartered Society of Physiotherapy, 1999). The prescription of muscle relaxants such as diazepam can be a useful adjunct to this physical therapy and break the vicious cycle between muscle spasm and pain. A variety of soft or rigid spinal braces may also be used to ease pain and facilitate earlier mobilisation. Long-term use of braces or supports is not recommended as muscle wasting and dependence develops.

Occupational therapists also play an important role in providing a variety of interventions to ease acute and chronic pain and to assist with the mobilization of osteoporotic patients in hospital and at home. Various aids may be required to enable the patient to manage their activities of daily living without exacerbating their pain.

4.3.4 **Osteoporosis treatment**

Pain control is the number one priority for patients presenting with acute and chronic pain due to osteoporosis. The fear of suffering further fractures is also of great importance.

The National Institute for Clinical Excellence (NICE) has published, and is currently reviewing, its guidance regarding the use of bisphosphonates, raloxifene, teriparatide, and strontium ranelate for osteoporotic fracture prevention in postmenopausal women (National Institute for Clinical Excellence, 2005). This guidance differs from the Royal College of Physicians Guidance (Royal College of Physicians, 2000). The expanding array of interventions for fracture prevention enable treatments to be tailored to the individual (Box 4.4).

If indicated, long-term oral bisphosphonates should be commenced as soon as possible in order to reduce the risks for further fractures (Black *et al.* 2000; Delmas *et al.* 2004; McClung *et al.* 2001). However

Box 4.4 Fracture prevention in osteoporosis

- Biphosphonates—alendronate, risedronate, etidronate, ibandronate, pamidronate
- Selective oestrogen receptor modulator—raloxifene
- Dual action bone agent—strontium ranelate
- Parathyroid hormone—teriparatide
- Adjuvant calcium and vitamin D supplementation
- Lifestyle modification—avoidance of tobacco use and alcohol abuse, regular weight bearing exercise, and adequate calcium intake.

these must not be started until the patient is able to comply with the administration instructions particularly with respect to remaining vertical (not necessarily standing!) for 30 minutes after ingestion. Patients must be informed that these drugs are prescribed to treat their osteoporosis not their pain. Patients receiving bisphosphonates must not be deficient in calcium and vitamin D and supplementation is often required for care home residents.

Raloxifene is currently recommended by NICE as an alternative treatment for secondary fracture prevention in patients who are intolerant of bisphosphonates, are unable to take them correctly or have failed to respond to them. However, this guidance is under review. NICE appraisal documents state that raloxifene is not cost effective for the primary prevention of osteoporotic fractures but this guidance is yet to be finalized.

Strontium ranelate is licensed for the treatment of post-menopausal women with osteoporosis and has shown to be beneficial even for the oldest patients. It is reported to reduce pain at the spine and improve quality of life (Meunier *et al.* 2004; Reginster *et al.* 2005). NICE are reviewing the role of strontium in both primary and secondary fracture prevention.

Subcutaneous parathyroid hormone therapy is currently limited by NICE to the treatment of older postmenopausal women with severe established osteoporosis who have failed to tolerate or respond to oral bisphosphonates and can be given for a maximum of 18 months only (Neer *et al.* 2001). There is less evidence and guidance for men with osteoporosis. Although treatment is similar, with the exception of raloxifene, it is generally recommended that advice from a specialized osteoporosis clinician is sought.

4.3.5 **Interventional radiology**

Vertebroplasty may be used for patients whose severe pain has failed to improve despite four to six weeks of conservative therapy. Under X-ray guidance, cement is injected into the body of the fractured vertebra. This is reported to give significant short-term pain relief, presumably by stabilizing the vertebra and possibly due to thermal necrosis of nerves by the hot cement. However there is no significant reduction in pain at 12 months compared to similar patients managed conservatively (Diamond *et al.* 2006). Kyphoplasty involves the insertion of a balloon into the vertebral body; this is inflated and filled with cement. It is believed that the structural support within the vertebra and correction of the deformity, contributes to the pain relief (Grafe *et al.* 2005). Serious complications have been reported with both of these procedures and they must only be performed in units that have the support of a spinal surgeon (National Institute for Clinical Excellence, 2003, 2006).

4.3.6 **Psychological support**

Psychological support is essential especially for those who are struggling to deal with their pain and are distressed by their new diagnosis of osteoporosis, altered body image, and loss of independence. The members of the multidisciplinary team will offer support to inpatients and outpatients. The expertise of a psychologist or psychiatrist may also be required and this is covered more fully in Chapter 9. Pain management clinics provide a wide variety of helpful interventions including advice on neuropathic agents such as amitryptiline and gabapentin, the whole spectrum of analgesics, nerve blocks, facet joint injections, and physical and psychological techniques for coping with pain.

Osteoporosis nurse specialists, in the hospital or community, deliver essential services to patients, carers, and health professionals. They may be involved at an early stage diagnosing and managing the osteoporosis following a fracture and making referrals to appropriate members of the multidisciplinary team for pain management. They also offer important lifestyle advice, supportive helplines, and links to the many external and charitable organizations that are available to older people with osteoporosis and their carers.

The National Osteoporosis Society has a wide range of resources available covering all aspects of the condition including how to cope after a fracture (National Osteoporosis Society, 2003).

4.4 Conclusion

Although osteoporosis often goes unnoticed for many years, it is clearly a condition that causes a great deal of suffering among older people. Underlying causes of low bone density must be excluded and fracture prevention therapy commenced according to current national guidelines and clinical indications. It is essential that the multifactorial acute and chronic pains associated with osteoporotic fractures and deformities are carefully assessed (Box 4.5).

Whilst much of the clinical guidance for managing osteoporosis focuses on fracture prevention rather than the complexities of pain control, the multidisciplinary team members have a wealth of experience to draw on and are able to provide very effective integrated pain management services for older people with osteoporosis (Box 4.6).

Box 4.5 Multifactorial pains of osteoporosis

Acute

- Fractured hip/pelvis/wrist/rib
- Fractured vertebra
- Muscle spasm
- Nerve root pain

Chronic

- Muscle spasm
- Nerve root pain
- Degenerative disc disease
- Secondary osteoarthritis of hip/knee/shoulders/spine
- Impingement of ribs and pelvis
- Deformity and ligament strain
- Functional impairment
- Depression

Box 4.6 Multidisciplinary team approach

- Analgesia titrated to need
- Orthopaedic or spinal surgery
- Orthogeriatric care
- Interventional radiology
- Physiotherapy
- Occupational therapy
- Chronic pain clinic support
- Psychological support
- Osteoporosis management
- Exclusion of other pathology
- Falls prevention

References

Black DM, Thompson DE, Bauer DC, *et al.* (2000). Fracture risk reduction with alendronate in women with osteoporosis: the Fracture Intervention Trial. FIT Research Group. *Journal of Clinical Endocrinology and Metabolism*, **85**(11), 4118–24.

Compston J. (2000). *Osteoporosis—clinical guidelines for prevention and treatment. Update on pharmacological interventions and an algorithm for management.* **34** Royal College of Physicians, London. www.replondon.ac.uk

Delmas PD, Recker RR, Chestnut CH, *et al.* (2004). Daily and intermittent ibandronate normalise bone turnover and provide significant reduction in vertebral fracture risk: results from the BONE study. *Osteoporosis International*, **15**(10), 792–8.

Diamond TH, Bryant C, Browne L, *et al.* (2006). Clinical outcomes after acute osteoporotic vertebral fractures: a 2-year non-randomised trial comparing percutaneous vertebraoplasty with conservative therapy. *Medical Journal of Australia*, **184**(3), 113–17.

Grafe IA, Da Fonseca K, Hillmeier J, *et al.* (2005). Reduction of pain and fracture incidence after kyphoplasty: 1-year outcomes of a prospective controlled trial of patients with primary osteoporosis. *Osteoporosis International*, **16**(12), 2005–12.

Knopp JA, Diner BM, Blitz M, *et al.* (2005). Calcitonin for treating acute pain of osteoporotic vertebral compression fractures: a systematic review of randomised controlled trials. *Osteoporosis International*, **16**(10), 1281–90.

Lips P and Van Schoor NM (2005). Quality of life in patients with osteoporosis. *Osteoporosis International*, **16**(5), 447–55.

Malmros B, Mortensen L, Jensen MB, *et al.* (1998). Positive effects of physiotherapy on chronic pain and performance in osteoporosis. *Osteoprosis International*, **8**(3), 215–21.

McClung MR, Geunsens P, Miller PD, *et al.* (2001). Effect of risedronate on the risk of hip fracture in elderly women. Hip Intervention Program Study Group. *New England Journal of Medicine*, **344**(5), 333–40.

Meunier PJ, Roux C, Seeman E, *et al.* (2004). The effects of strontium ranelate on the risk of vertebral fracture in women with osteoporosis. *New England Journal of Medicine*, **350**(5), 459–68.

Mitchell SL, Creed G, Thow M, *et al.* (1999). *Physiotherapy Guidelines for the Management of Osteoporosis.* Chartered Society of Physiotherapists, London. www.csp.org.uk/uploads/documents/OSTEOgl.pdf

Morrison RS, Chassin MR, Siu AL, *et al.* (1998). The medical consultant's role in caring for patients with hip fracture. *Annals of Internal Medicine*, **128**(12), 1010–20.

Morrison RS, Magaziner J, Mclaughlin MA, *et al.* (2003). The impact of post-operative pain on outcomes following hip fracture. *Pain*, **103**(3), 303–11.

NICE (2003). *Percutaneous Vertebroplasty.* Interventional Procedure Guidance 12. National Institute for Clinical Excellence, London. www.nice.org.uk/guidance/IPG12

NICE (2005). *Bisphosphonates (alendronate, etidronate, risedronate), selective oestrogen receptor modulators (raloxifene) and parathyroid hormone (teriparatide) for the secondary prevention of osteoporotic fragility fractures in post menopausal women.* Technology Appraisal Guidance 87. National Institute for Clinical Excellence, London. www.nice.org.uk/guidance/TA87

NICE (2006). *Balloon Kyphoplasty for vertebral compression fractures.* Interventional Procedure Guidance 166. National Institute for Health and Clinical Excellence, London. www.nice.org.uk/download-aspx?0=1PG166publicinfo

National Osteoporosis Society (2003). *Living with Osteoporosis. Coping after broken bones.* National Osteoporosis Society, Bath. www.nos.org.uk

Neer RM, Arnaud CD, Zanchetta JR, *et al.* (2001). Effect of parathyroid hormone (1–34) on fractures and bone mineral density in postmenopausal women with osteoporosis. *New England Journal of Medicine,* **344**(19), 1434–41.

Reginster JY, Seeman E, De Vernejoul MC, *et al.* (2005). Strontium ranelate reduces the risk of nonvertebral fractures in postmenopausal women with osteoporosis: Treatment of Peripheral Osteoporosis (TROPOS) study. *Journal of Clinical Endocrinology and Metabolism,* **90**(50), 2816–22.

Roche JJW, Wenn RT, Sahota O, *et al.* (2005). Effects of comorbidities and postoperative complications on mortality after hip fracture in elderly people: prospective observational cohort study. *British Medical Journal,* **331**, (7529) 1374–6. Originally published online 18 November 2005, doi: 10.1136/bmj.38643.663843.55

Venning G (2005). Recent developments in Vitamin D deficiency and muscle weakness among elderly people. *British Medical Journal,* **330**, 524–6.

WHO (1994). *Assessment of fracture risk and its application to screening for postmenopausal osteoporosis.* World Health Organization Technical Report Series 843. World Health Organization, Geneva. www.who.int/reproductive-health/publications/abstracts/osteoporosis.html

Chapter 5

Musculoskeletal pain

Karen Walker-Bone

Key points

- Musculoskeletal pain is common amongst the elderly.
- It can be the presenting feature of malignant disease and careful clinical assessment is mandatory.
- Osteoarthritis, osteoporosis, rheumatoid arthritis, gout, pseudogout, polymyalgia rheumatica, and giant cell arteritis are the musculoskeletal conditions most likely to present among the elderly (aged over 50 years).
- Pain management should be tailored appropriately to the underlying diagnosis with simple and safe interventions first.

5.1 Introduction

Pain from the musculoskeletal system is common at all ages, but increases markedly with age (Badley & Tennant, 1992). The severity of joint symptoms also increases with age and the prevalence of associated disability increases steeply with age: according to one study, only 10% of those aged 16–34 years with joint symptoms reported disability, but this increased to 90% of subjects with joint pains aged over 85 years (Badley & Tennant, 1992). Indeed, musculoskeletal disorders account for half of all chronic disease among adults aged over 65 years. Given the expected worldwide demographic changes, the World Health Organization project that osteoarthritis will be the disease associated with the 4th most significant impact among women and 8th among men by 2020 (Murray & Lopez, 1997).

Musculoskeletal pain can be attributed to a wide diversity of pathologies (Box 5.1). Importantly however, musculoskeletal pain may be the presenting feature of malignant disease, especially among older people. Accordingly, the assessment of all older people presenting with musculoskeletal symptoms should always include a thorough history and examination and appropriate use of clinical investigations. Figure 5.1 summarizes the Clinical Standards Advisory

Box 5.1 Musculoskeletal pathologies

- Soft tissue regional pain syndromes e.g. back pain and neck pain
- Generalized soft tissue pain syndromes e.g. fibromyalgia syndrome
- Osteoarthritis
- Osteoporosis
- Inflammatory arthritis e.g. rheumatoid arthritis, gout
- Generalized inflammatory conditions e.g. polymyalgia rheumatica, connective tissue diseases

Figure 5.1 'Red flags' for the assessment of back pain (adapted from Murray, 1997)

Red flags in back pain

- Age of onset <20 or >55 years
- Violent trauma (fracture)
- Unrelenting pain (not positional, increasing with time, day and night)
- Objective neurological disturbance, muscle wasting or weakness, bladder or bowel control affected
- General ill health: weight loss, fever, night sweats
- Neurological symptoms or signs
- Thoracic pain
- Past history of carcinoma
- Structural deformity
- Lumbar flexion consistently restricted
- Immunosuppression of any cause
- Systemic corticosteroids

Group (1994) recommended 'red flags' for the assessment of back pain which provide useful general principles for the assessment of any new presentation of musculoskeletal pain.

5.2 Osteoarthritis

5.2.1 Epidemiology

Osteoarthritis (OA) is a common, chronic, musculoskeletal disorder. Symptomatic OA, particularly of the knee and hip, is the most common cause of musculoskeletal disability in the elderly (Felson *et al.* 1987).

Radiologists and pathologists coined the term 'osteoarthritis' originally, to describe the appearances of overgrowth of the marginal and subchondral bone. Pathologically, the dominant process is that of focal destruction of articular cartilage, accompanied by a hypertrophic reaction at the joint margins and in the subchondral bone. The current view of OA is that it represents a heterogeneous group of overlapping pathological conditions, causing damage to the articular cartilage and leading to clinically and radiographically recognized impairment of the joints and disability of the patient.

5.2.2 **Clinical features**

OA results in painful stiff joints with limited movement. The pain of osteoarthritis tends to worsen on use and may often occur at night after a period of rest. Joint stiffness also increases with inactivity and may occur at night but should not last longer than 30 minutes (in contrast with the stiffness associated with inflammatory arthritis). Some individuals develop a characteristic pattern of joint involvement, affecting the hands (distal interphalangeal joints, proximal interphalangeal joints, and 1st carpometacarpal joints), hips, knees, and spine symmetrically; this pattern is often familial.

5.2.3 **Clinical assessment**

The main reasons for which an OA patient seeks medical help are pain and functional impairment. However, the correlation between pain severity, disability, and structural changes is poor and the consequences of pain and impairment on individuals vary dependent upon their personality, affect, occupation, psychosocial environment, and expectations (Brandt *et al.* 1998). Investigations should include inflammatory markers (erthrocyte sedimentation rate (ESR)/C-reactive protein (CRP), which should be normal, and radiographs of affected joints.

5.2.4 **Clinical management**

SIMPLE and SAFE interventions should be utilized first (Figures. 5.2 and 5.3): education, social support, physiotherapy (both specific muscle strengthening and general fitness), occupational therapy, acupuncture and transcutaneous electrical nerve stimulation (TENS) are non-pharmacological therapies with established evidence-based efficacy (Pendleton *et al.* 2000).

Pharmacological therapies are utilized as second-line therapy (Figure 7.1, Chapter 7) for uncontrolled pain. The results of meta-analyses have shown evidence for the safety and effectiveness of topical non-steroidal anti-inflammatory drugs in osteoarthritis (Pendleton *et al.* 2000). Topical capsaicin, the natural substance found inside the white 'ribs' of hot chilli peppers and responsible for the familiar 'burning' sensation, reversibly depletes substance P. A meta-analysis concluded that capsaicin was useful in the treatment of OA with

Figure 5.2 Management of osteoarthritis of the first carpo-metacarpophalangeal joint

OA of the 1st CMCJ

Pragmatic management algorithm

1. Check correct diagnosis (ESR normal, X-ray changes)
2. Topical NSAIDs
3. Topical capsaicin
4. Simple analgesics
5. Oral NSAIDs/COX-2 inhibitors
6. Local corticosteroid injection
7. Surgery

Figure 5.3 Management of osteoarthritis of the knee (Walker-Bone *et al.*, 2000)

OA of the knee

Pragmatic management algorithm

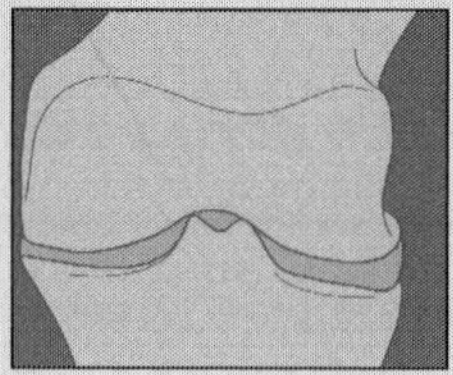

1. Check correct diagnosis (ESR normal, X-ray changes)
2. Topical NSAIDs
3. Simple analgesics
4. Oral NSAIDs/COX-2 inhibitors
5. Local corticosteroid injection
6. Hyaluronan/tidal irrigation
7. Arthroscopic washout/surgery

odds ratio in favour of capsaicin over placebo of 4.36 (Zhang & Li-Wan-Po, 1994). However, placebo-controlled trials with this agent, which causes pronounced burning, are understandably difficult and most studies show profoundly positive effects of topical placebo.

Paracetamol in doses up to 4g/day is safe and effective in OA (Pendleton *et al.* 2000). When paracetamol is compared to non-steroidal anti-inflammatory drugs (NSAIDs), none of the assessed outcomes (pain at rest, pain on motion, walking time over 50 feet, and quality of life measures) showed a significant advantage of the NSAIDs over simple analgesics. However, there were high rates of dropout in all studies, suggesting that neither NSAIDs nor simple analgesics are totally effective at relieving the pain of OA. There was some evidence to suggest a slight benefit of the addition of dextropropoxyphene to paracetamol, but coproxamol has been recently withdrawn in the UK after concerns about safety (Duff 2005).

Despite an absence of long-term data, and short-term studies that show advantage for NSAIDs over placebo but have high drop out rates, NSAIDs have remained a popular choice for the management of OA. NSAIDs are still persistently prescribed as first-line therapy and many patients purchase ibuprofen over the counter. Against this backdrop, the COX-2 inhibitors were marketed in the late 1990s. Short-term studies demonstrating comparable pain-relieving properties in arthritis patients (Bombardier *et al.* 2000), but with a 50% reduction in endoscopic ulceration (Bombardier *et al.* 2000), led to a rapid proliferation in prescriptions for OA (Shaughnessy & Gordon, 2006). However, the cardiovascular safety of rofecoxib was questioned soon after licensing and the drug was withdrawn by its manufacturers in 2005, amidst study results suggesting a significantly increased risk of cardiovascular disease (Shaughnessy & Gordon, 2006). Recently, studies have questioned the cardiovascular safety of conventional NSAIDs and 'traditional' OA drugs such as diclofenac and ibuprofen have been implicated in increased susceptibility to cardiovascular disease (Kearney *et al.* 2006). Pragmatically, there is little evidence to support the long-term efficacy of either NSAIDs or COX-2 inhibitors for the pain of OA and, whilst there is considerable uncertainty about the cardiovascular safety of these pharmacological interventions, they are best reserved as third-line therapies, prescribed only after assessment of cardiovascular risk factors.

The 'Holy Grail' for OA remains the challenge of finding agents with chondroprotective properties. To date, there has been no convincing evidence from human studies that chondroprotection could even be achieved, but there have been data from animal studies, and the emergence of glucosamine sulphate, chondroitin sulphate, avocado and soya unsaponifiables, diaceirin, and hyaluronic acid have suggested that, theoretically, cartilage damage could be preventable. In particular, initial studies with glucosamine sulphate and chondroitin sulphate showed promise but more recent studies have failed to show significant effect (Clegg *et al.* 2006; McAlindon, 2006).

Intra-articular corticosteroids are frequently used in OA, particularly in a joint with significant effusion or other signs of inflammation. There are several small randomized controlled trials that confirm the short-term efficacy of this approach (Walker-Bone *et al.* 2000). However, this approach usually represents a palliation in OA. Should symptoms recur, referral for arthroscopy and/or surgery would usually be considered unless the patient is medically unfit for surgical intervention.

5.3 Inflammatory arthritis

5.3.1 Rheumatoid arthritis

5.3.1.1 *Epidemiology*

Around 387,000 adults in the UK have rheumatoid arthritis (RA), the most common form of inflammatory arthritis. It affects around three times as many women as men and can present at any age with age-adjusted incidence rates of 0.1–0.7/1000 patient years at risk (Arthritis and Musculoskeletal Alliance, 2004).

5.3.1.2 *Clinical features*

RA is a symmetrical polyarthritis affecting any synovial joint. It commonly causes stiffness, which is most severe on waking and can last several hours before mobility increases. Joints are painful, warm, swollen, and, if untreated, become deformed in characteristic patterns. Systemic, non-articular manifestations are common (Box 5.2).

Box 5.2 Systemic, non-articular manifestations

- Normocytic, normochromic anaemia
- Fatigue
- Malaise
- Weight loss
- Nodules
- Vasculitis
- Pericarditis and pulmonary fibrosis
- Hepatosplenomegaly
- Neurological including cord compression and peripheral nerve lesions
- Ocular involvement including Sjogren's syndrome
- Panyctopenia and lymphadenopathy (Felty's syndrome)
- Renal disease including amyloidosis

5.3.1.3 *Clinical assessment*

The diagnosis of RA is made from a variety of clinical features and investigation findings (Table 5.1).

5.3.1.4 *Clinical management*

The principles of management rely upon providing rapid relief of pain and symptoms and long-term disease suppression to prevent disease progression, deformity, and disability. Short-term relief may be achieved with analgesics and/or NSAIDs. Glucocorticoids also have established efficacy, bring rapid relief and may have beneficial disease modification properties in the first 12 months after diagnosis (Machold *et al.* 2006). Long-term disease modification is achieved with disease-modifying anti-rheumatic drugs (DMARDs), which may be used in combination, or with the anti-tumour necrosis factor (anti-TNF) therapies (Table 5.2) (Walker-Bone & Farrow, 2006).

Table 5.1 American College of Rheumatology Diagnostic criteria for Rheumatoid Arthritis (Arnett *et al.* 1988)

Criterion	Definition
1. Morning stiffness	Morning stiffness in and around the joints lasting at least 1 hour before maximal improvement. At least 3 joints
2. Arthritis of 3 or more joint areas	Areas simultaneously have had soft tissue swelling or fluid (not just bony overgrowth) observed by a physician
3. Arthritis of hand joints	At least one area swollen in a wrist, MCP or PIP joint with soft tissue swelling or fluid at the interview, or deformity and a documented history of swelling
4. Symmetrical arthritis	Simultaneous involvement of the same joint areas on both sides of the body (bilateral movement of PIPs, MCPs, or MTPs is acceptable without absolute symmetry)
5. Rheumatoid nodules	Subcutaneous nodules, over bony prominences, or extensor or extra-articular regions, observed by a physician
6. Serum rheumatoid factor	Demonstration of abnormal amounts of serum rheumatoid factor by any method for which the results have been positive for less than 5% of control subjects
7. Radiographic changes	Radiographic changes typical of RA on posteroanterior hand and wrist radiographs, which must include erosions or unequivocal bone decalcification localized in or most marked adjacent to the involved joint

5.3.2 **Gout**

5.3.2.1 ***Epidemiology***

Gout is the most common cause of inflammatory arthritis in men aged over 40 years and is rare in children and premenopausal women (Jordan, 2004). In the UK, the prevalence was estimated as 2.6/1000 in both genders combined for persons aged over 15 years. Prevalence was greater among men than women and increased with age. The annual incidence of gout among UK men has been estimated as 7.6/1000 and among UK women as 2.5/1000 over the age of 75 years (Stewart & Silman, 1990). The key risk factor for gout is sustained hyperuricaemia, but gout is also associated with obesity, alcohol intake, hypertension, and exposure to raised levels of lead. Hyperuricaemia and gout may represent another marker of the metabolic syndrome (central obesity, hypertension, hyperlipidaemia, glucose intolerance) and increased risk of cardiovascular disease. Hyperuricaemia also predisposes to nephrolithiasis.

Table 5.2 DMARDS and anti-TNF agents commonly used in RA

DMARDs	**Properties**
Methotrexate	Gold standard usually first-line therapy. Administered orally weekly.
Sulfasalazine	Other choice of first-line therapy. Administered orally daily.
Leflunomide	Second-line therapy. Administered orally daily.
Azathioprine	Second-line therapy. Administered orally daily.
Hydroxychloroquine	Used for mild disease or in combination with methotrexate and sulfasalazine.
Cyclosporine	Second-line therapy. Administered orally daily.
Gold salts	Second- or third-line therapy. Administered parenterally weekly initially.
D-penicillamine	Second- or third-line therapy. Administered orally daily.
Anti-TNF agents	**Properties**
Infliximab	Administered by intravenous infusion 8-weekly after original dose-loading.
Etanercept	Administered by subcutaneous injection 50mg weekly or 25mg twice weekly.
Adalimumab	Administered by subcutaneous injection fortnightly.

5.3.2.2 *Clinical features*

The clinical history is the most likely clue to the diagnosis. Classically, there is a relatively rapid onset of pain in the relevant part, such as the big toe joint, often in the early hours of the morning. The part becomes hot, red, and very tender, so that even bedclothes may be too heavy. 50% of first attacks and 70% of all gout attacks occur in the big toe ('podagra'). The affected joint is warm, swollen, and tender and adjacent skin is often erythematous. An attack of gout may be accompanied by a systemic inflammatory response. Acute attacks rarely last more than two weeks, even without treatment and there may be a prolonged duration between attacks.

5.3.2.3 *Clinical assessment*

The most important differential diagnosis of acute gout is infective arthritis. A systemic inflammatory reaction may be demonstrated on blood tests with elevated ESR and CRP and a mild neutrophil leucocytosis. Serum uric acid cannot be used as a diagnostic test as urate

Table 5.3 Therapies for chronic gout (Stewart & Silman, 1990)	
Mechanism of Action	**Names of drugs**
Uricostatic	Xanthine oxidase inhibitors e.g. allopurinol, oxipurinol. New agent entering clinical trials in the UK: febuxostat
Uricosuric	e.g. benzbromarone, sulfinpyrazone, probenecid
Uricolytic	e.g urate oxidase

levels frequently decrease during an acute attack. Imaging, particularly plain X-rays are unhelpful acutely but can be helpful in chronic tophaceous gout. The only unequivocal way of confirming the diagnosis is by aspirating the affected joint, and demonstrating typically shaped negatively birefringent crystals on polarized light microscopy (monosodium urate crystals).

5.3.2.4 ***Clinical management***

An acute attack should be terminated as rapidly as possible with rest and pharmacological interventions. Treatment options include NSAIDs, colchicine, and glucocorticoids (systemic or intra-articular). Urate-lowering drugs should be continued throughout an acute episode if commenced previously, but should not be commenced during an acute attack (Jordan, 2004). Once an attack is controlled, the aim is to prevent subsequent attacks by combining lifestyle modification (weight loss, diet (low purine), alcohol reduction/cessation, avoiding diuretic therapy) with pharmacological therapy (Table 5.3).

5.3.3 **Pseudogout/calcium pyrophosphate dehydrate deposition disease (CPPD)**

5.3.3.1 ***Epidemiology***

These are a number of heterogeneous conditions with linked pathological, radiological, and clinical features. The pathology is deposition of calcium salt crystals, predominantly calcium phosphate, but also including hydroxyapatite. 'Pseudogout' was attributed to these conditions in the 1960s, as they cause acute arthritis with a presentation similar to gout in the absence of uric acid crystals (Dieppe, 2000). Given the heterogeneity of the underlying pathology, epidemiological study is complex. Pseudogout is rare in young people and increases in frequency with age, being the commonest cause of acute arthritis among those aged over 70 years. Women are slightly more commonly affected than men.

5.3.3.2 *Clinical features*

Pseudogout presents usually as an acute monoarthritis. The knee is by far the commonest joint affected by attacks. The wrist, shoulder, ankle, and elbow are the other joints that are most likely to be involved. Attacks are almost always confined to a single joint. Typically, one joint develops intense pain and swelling with increasing severity over 6–24 hours of onset. Systemic fever may be associated. If untreated, an attack may take 2–3 weeks to resolve. Some patients experience only one attack during a lifetime, but others experience recurrent attacks.

5.3.3.3 *Clinical assessment*

The diagnosis may be strongly suggested by the history, particularly, for example, in the case of a monoarthritis of the knee presenting in an elderly woman after an operation (Dieppe, 2000). The main differential diagnosis is septic arthritis. Blood tests may show a systemic inflammatory reaction (elevated ESR and CRP). Aspiration of the joint and demonstration of the positively birefringent crystals under polarized light microscopy is diagnostic and demonstration of radiological evidence of chondrocalcinosis in the affected joint is helpful.

5.3.3.4 *Clinical management*

The acute attack is managed with rest, NSAIDs, colchicine, and analgesia. Once the diagnosis is confirmed, and septic arthritis excluded, intra-articular glucocorticoids in the affected joint can be rapidly effective.

5.3.4 **Polymyalgia rheumatica and giant cell arteritis**

5.3.4.1 *Epidemiology*

Polymyalgia rheumatica (PMR) and giant cell arteritis (GCA) are two related disorders which may represent ends of a spectrum of systemic inflammatory rheumatic disorders of unknown aetiology. PMR is a relatively ill-defined clinical syndrome of limb girdle pain and stiffness in association with systemic features such as malaise, fever, and elevated inflammatory markers (ESR and CRP). GCA is a vasculitic disorder, which can be widely disseminated, affecting the medium and large arteries. The disorders frequently overlap so that series suggest that 20–30% of patients have features of both diseases. Both disorders become more frequent with age, and incidence rates range from 1–30/100,000 population aged over 50 years for GCA and 10–110/100,000 population aged over 50 years for PMR (Silman, 2001).

5.3.4.2 *Clinical features*

The patient (usually aged over 50 years) presents with non-specific symptoms (malaise, weight loss), feels unwell, and reports symmetrical pain and stiffness of the proximal muscle girdles. GCA is associated with localized severe headache, jaw claudication, scalp tenderness, and visual disturbance.

5.3.4.3 *Clinical Assessment*

The diagnostic criteria for GCA (Box 5.3) and PMR (Box 5.4) are shown. The diagnoses rely upon clinical features, laboratory investigation and biopsy of the temporal artery in suspected GCA.

5.3.4.4 *Clinical management*

GCA is an emergency, since it can be associated with rapid visual loss. Once suspected, high-dose oral glucocorticoids should be commenced immediately (60–80mg/day prednisolone). A rapid response is expected (within 48 hours). PMR not associated with GCA should be treated with conservative doses of glucocorticoids (maximum 15mg/day of prednisolone). The highest doses should be maintained for the first 12 weeks or so and then gradual reduction should be initiated to find the lowest dose that best controls clinical symptoms. Inflammatory markers (ESR/CRP) can be used for monitoring the effectiveness of therapy.

Box 5.3 American College of Rheumatology criteria for GCA (Hunder *et al.* 1990). The patient has to meet at least 3 of the 5 criteria

1. Age onset at least 50 years
2. New onset of localized headache (different from previous headache)
3. Tenderness or decreased pulsation in at least one of the temporal arteries
4. ESR $\geq$ 50mm/hour
5. Abnormal artery biopsy with either mononuclear cell infiltrate or granulomatous inflammation (with giant cells)

Box 5.4 UK criteria for PMR (Bird *et al.* 1979). The patient has to meet at least 3 of the 7 criteria

1. Bilateral shoulder pain and/or stiffness
2. Delay from onset to maximal symptoms <2 weeks
3. Initial ESR $\geq$40mm/hour
4. Morning stiffness >1 hour
5. Age over 65 years
6. Depression and/or loss of weight
7. Upper arm tenderness bilaterally

5.4 Soft tissue regional pain syndromes

A detailed description of these conditions is outside the scope of this chapter but, e.g., neck pain, knee pain, back pain are common symptoms at all ages. In the older patient, OA is a common contributing factor. However, it should be borne in mind that regional and widespread musculoskeletal pain may be the presenting feature of malignancy and a thorough evaluation of the history, examination, and basic investigations should be carried out, especially when symptoms are unrelenting after 4–6 weeks or 'red flags' are present (Figure 5.1).

5.5 Conclusion

Musculoskeletal pain is common at all ages, but is much more frequent in older patients. Some conditions are unlikely except in older patients: PMR, GCA, osteoporosis, and OA. A vigilant approach should be taken to the assessment of musculoskeletal symptoms in older patients, as non-specific symptoms and pain may be the presenting feature of severe or life-threatening conditions such as malignancy, myeloma, or vasculitis. A rheumatological assessment may be indicated in any patient who is failing to respond to analgesics and/or physiotherapy over 2–3 months.

References

Arnett FC, Edworthy SM, Bloch DA, *et al.* (1988). The American Rheumatism Association 1987 revised criteria for the classification of rheumatoid arthritis. *Arthritis Rheum*, **31**, 315–24.

Arthritis and Musculoskeletal Alliance (2004). *Standards of care for people with inflammatory arthritis.* ARMA London.

Badley EM and Tennant A (1992). Changing profile of joint disorders with age: findings from a postal survey of the population of Calderdale, West Yorkshire, United Kingdom. *Ann Rheum Dis*, **51**, 366–71.

Bird HA, Esselinckx W, Dixon AJ, *et al.* (1979). An evaluation of criteria for polymyalgia rheumatica. *Ann Rheum Dis*, **38**, 434–9.

Bombardier C, Laine L, Reicin A, *et al.* (2000). Comparison of upper gastrointestinal toxicity of rofecoxib and naproxen in patients with rheumatoid arthritis. *N Engl J Med*, **343**, 1520–8.

Brandt K, Lohmander LS, and Doherty M (1998). Management of osteoarthritis: Introduction, the comprehensive approach. In Brandt KD, Doherty M, and Lohmander LS (eds). *Osteoarthritis.* Oxford Medical Publications, Oxford. pp.250–5.

Clegg DO, Reda DJ, Harris CL, *et al.* (2006). Glucosamine, chondroitin sulfate, and the two in combination for painful knee osteoarthritis. *New Engl J Med*, **354**, 795–808.

Dieppe P (2000). Pseudogout-what's in a name? *Arthritis Research Campaign News & Features*, October. Chesterfield, UK. www.arc.org.uk/newsviews/arctdy/110/pseudog.htm

Duff G (2005). Withdrawal of co-proxamol products and interim updated prescribing information. In *Medicines and Healthcare Products Regulatory Agency*. Available online. URL: http://www.mhra.gov.uk/

Felson DT, Naimark A, Anderson JJ, *et al.* (1987). The prevalence of knee osteoarthritis in the elderly: The Framingham Osteoarthritis Study. *Arthritis Rheum*, **30**, 914–18.

Hunder GG, Bloch DA, Michel BA, *et al.* (1990). The American college of rheumatology 1990 criteria for the classification of giant cell arteritis. *Arthritis Rheum*, **33**, 1122–8.

Jordan K (2004). *An update on gout.* Topical Reviews: Reports on the Rheumatic Diseases series 5. Arthritis Research Campaign, Chesterfield, UK.

Kearney PM, Baigent C, Godwin J, *et al.* (2006). Do selective cyclo-oxygenase-2 inhibitors and traditional non-steroidal anti-inflmmatory drugs increase the risk of atherothrombosis? Meta-analysis of randomized trials. *BMJ*, **332**, 1302–8.

McAlindon TE (2006). Nutraceuticals: do they work and when should we use them? *Best Pract Res Clin Rheumatol*, **20**, 99–115.

Machold KP, Nell V, Stamm T, *et al.* (2006). Early rheumatoid arthritis. *Curr Opin Rheumatol*, **18**, 282–8.

Murray CJL and Lopez AD (1997). *The global burden of disease.* World Health Organization, Geneva.

Pendleton A, *et al.* (2000). *Ann Rheum Dis*, **59**, 936–44.

Report of a Clinical Standards Advisory Group Committee on Back Pain, Chair Prof. Michael Rosen (May 1994). *Back pain.* HMSO, London.

Shaughnessy AF and Gordon AE (2006). Life without COX-2 inhibitors. *BMJ*, **332**, 1287–8.

Silman AJ (2001). Polymyalgia rheumatica and giant cell arteritis. In Silman AJ, Hochberg M (eds.), *Epidemiology of the rheumatic diseases*, second edition. Oxford University Press, Oxford pp.188–204.

Stewart OJ and Silman AJ (1990). Review of the Uk data on the rheumatic diseases-4. Gout. *Br J Rheumatol*, **29**, 485–8.

Walker-Bone K, Javaid K, Arden N, *et al.* (2000). The medical management of osteoarthritis. *BMJ*, **321**, 936–40.

Walker-Bone K and Farrow S. Rheumatoid arthritis; Clinical evidence (In press).

Zhang WY and Li-Wan-Po A (1994). The effectiveness of topically applied capsaicin. A meta-analysis. *Eur J Clin Pharmacol*, **46**, 517–22.

Chapter 6

Abdominal pain

Krishna Moorthy and Mark Deakin

Key points

- Diagnosis of a cause for abdominal pain is based on the site and characteristics of the pain together with a knowledge of likely pathology.
- For foregut pathology pain is epigastric.
- For midgut pathology pain is central (peri-umbilical).
- For hindgut pathology pain is in the lower abdomen.
- Once there is inflammation, pain and tenderness become localized to the abdominal wall overlying the organ concerned.

6.1 The clinical problem

Abdominal pain is a common clinical problem at all ages although with advancing years the likelihood of serious intra-abdominal pathology increases. Biliary disease in combination with gallstones is extremely common and the peak incidence of tumours of the stomach, pancreas and colon is between 60–70 years old. Diverticular disease of the colon and its complications are also extremely common but some diseases including appendicitis and perforated duodenal ulcer are less common in older patients.

In an ageing population who are still relatively fit it is common to get two or more coexisting significance pathologies (Hilliard *et al.* 2004). Thus, for example, pain from a right-sided colon cancer may be ascribed to incidental gallstones or diverticular disease.

6.2 Pathophysiology of abdominal pain

The differential diagnosis of the cause of any abdominal pain is based on site, onset, character, radiation, exacerbating and relieving factors, and a knowledge of the most likely underlying pathology.

Pain signals from an intra-abdominal organ are transmitted via autonomic afferents to the dorsal root ganglion of the spinal cord which also receives somatic afferents from the relevant dermatome.

Such pain that arises in intra-abdominal organs but is perceived in a corresponding somatic dermatome is called **referred pain**. This pain is poorly localized but felt more generally. For foregut structures, pain is felt in the epigastrium via the greater splanchnic nerves to the T5–9 dermatomes; for midgut structures in the centre of the abdomen–peri-umbilical area via the lesser splanchnic nerves; or for the hindgut structures in the lower abdomen or hypogastrium via the least splanchnic nerves (Figure 6.1).

Figure 6.1 Schematic representation of the referred site of abdominal pain

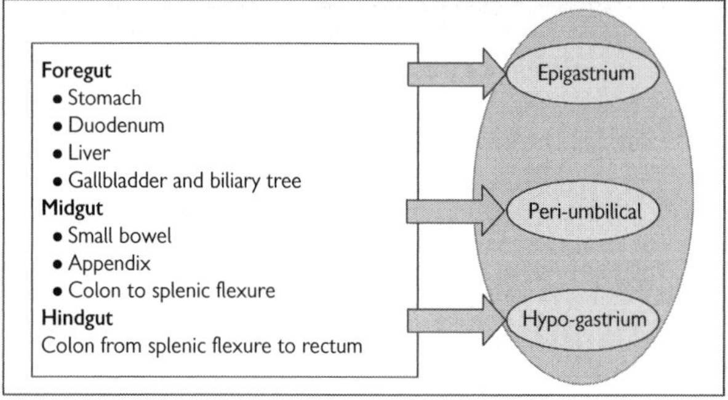

The peritoneal nerve supply corresponds to that of the overlying area of abdominal wall. Therefore, once inflammation of an organ affects the adjacent peritoneum, pain and tenderness become localized. The only exception to this is where diaphragmatic irritation causes pain to be felt in the shoulder tip. This is because the phrenic nerve which innervates the diaphragm shares the same nerve roots as the cutaneous supply to this area (C4).

The classical example of **shifting pain** is that of appendicitis where visceral pain from the appendix, a midgut structure, is initially felt around the umbilicus or centrally in the abdomen. This pain is initially poorly localized. When the inflammation subsequently affects the peritoneum in the right iliac fossa overlying the appendix, the pain then **shifts** to that area and tenderness becomes more localized. Similarly, once a patient develops diverticulitis of the sigmoid colon, initially poorly localized pain in the lower abdomen becomes localized tenderness and guarding in the left iliac fossa as inflammation of the overlying parietal peritoneum develops.

Since the possible causes of abdominal pain are legion it is best to consider some common presentations and their differential diagnoses.

6.3 Upper abdominal pain

Box 6.1 Case study A

Mrs Jones, a 79-year-old previously well lady presents with a six-month history of intermittent colicky, right hypochondrial/epigastric pain radiating to the back. Episodes occur two to three times a week lasting from 30 minutes to several hours at a time, often related to meals. The pain is often associated with vomiting which she finds relieves her pain.

6.3.1 Diagnosis and management

The diagnosis here is likely to be biliary colic in association with gallstones. Up to 10% of the older population have gallstones although nearly two-thirds of these are asymptomatic (Halldestam *et al.* 2004). Since gallstones are so common it is important not to assume that they are the cause of the pain unless the history is characteristic. The diagnosis is made clinically supported by ultrasound examination. The things to look for on the ultrasound report are the presence of gallstones in the gallbladder and the thickness of the gallbladder wall which if thickened would suggest that there has been previous cholecystitis. In this instance there would typically have been a history of previous pyrexia in association with one of the attacks and the likelihood of a more prolonged episode of right upper quadrant abdominal tenderness. Whether the bile duct is dilated or not is also important as this might suggest that there are bile duct stones. It is also important to check the liver function tests to consider the possibility of bile duct stones, in which case there may be a history of intermittent jaundice or cholangitis. In this instance, characteristically, alkaline phosphatase and gamma glutamyl transferase levels would be elevated rather than the transaminases.

Management of gallstones is by either conservative measures of low fat, high fibre diets, simple analgesics, and possibly an anti-spasmodic during attacks. If these attacks are occurring more frequently than is acceptable to the patient, frequently interfering with lifestyle and often so bad that the patient says 'I never want to go through that pain again', then the only effective treatment option is to consider cholecystectomy. Other non-operative options such as gallstone dissolution therapy and lithotripsy have poor long-term results. Occasionally, in unfit patients having severe problems, percutaneous gallstone extraction can be performed under local anaesthetic. Laparoscopic cholecystectomy however is a very safe option with low risk of perioperative morbidity and mortality and early return to normal function, even in older patients (Bingener *et al.* 2003). Thus the main indication for surgery is prevention of recurrent bouts of biliary colic or cholecystitis. If symptoms are due to complications such as stone migration into the CBD, gallstone pancreatitis, cholangitis, or cholestasis then these stones can be removed at ERCP (endoscopic retrograde cholangio-pancreatography). In this instance the incidence of subsequent problems related to the gallbladder itself is approximately 15% in older patients so the gallbladder can be left insitu (Pring *et al.* 2005).

6.3.2 **Differential diagnosis**

Oesophageal pain from reflux can also be felt in the epigastrium which tends to be a characteristic burning pain (heartburn), extremely common as over 10% of the population experience reflux type problems (Blustein *et al.* 1998). Symptoms are most often felt post-prandially or when the patient is supine and associated features such as regurgitation are common. Response to treatment with a proton pump inhibitor is usually satisfactory and is virtually a diagnostic test of an acid related disorder.

Similar burning epigastric pain can be due to both gastric and duodenal ulceration which fortunately is currently less common. Both are still seen relatively commonly in association with both steroids and non-steroidal anti-inflammatory drugs but prophylaxis with misoprostol or a proton pump inhibitor in this situation has reduced the incidence of problems. In gastric ulcers pain may occur soon after food and is associated with vomiting. Patients are generally reluctant to eat. Pain from duodenal ulcers occurs 2–3 hours after a meal and is relieved by food (hunger pains). Treatment again is by the use of proton pump inhibitors in association with eradication of *Helicobacter pylori* if present on faecal antigen testing. *H. pylori* testing and treatment can be used as a 'test and treat' option for characteristic acid-peptic pain although it should be remembered that *H. pylori* is present in a significant percentage of the population incidentally.

Unfortunately gastric malignancy can present in a similar way, and **all new onset dyspepsia** in the elderly, especially if associated with alarm symptoms (weight loss, loss of appetite, anaemia, haemetemesis/malaena, persistent vomiting, mass in the abdomen), should be investigated by endoscopy (National Institute of Clinical Excellence guidelines, 2004a). Once there is associated weight loss and a palpable abdominal mass then the cancer is almost certainly incurable. Stage for stage, results of gastric resection in older patients are equivalent to those of younger patients but will depend on associated comorbidity.

Most pancreatic cancers are located in the head of the gland and most often presents classically with painless obstructive jaundice. Pancreatic pain is often felt in the mid-back and can be a chronic unremitting problem. When pain occurs, para-aortic lymph node involvement is common and is a poor prognostic sign Chronic pancreatitis is an uncommon diagnosis in the elderly unless there has been a preceding history of earlier pancreatic problems or alcohol abuse.

Hepatic pain is also felt in the epigastrium. Presentation in older patients with liver metastases from an intra-abdominal source (colon or pancreas most commonly) is possible. Liver function tests are usually elevated; tumour markers can be helpful in identifying a possible site of primary. Initial investigation is by ultrasound examination followed by CT scan.

6.4 Central abdominal pain

Box 6.2 Case study B

Mr West, a 75-year-old, presents acutely with a 24-hour history of colicky central abdominal pain and vomiting. Abdominal examination shows that he has a distended abdomen and that there is mild generalized tenderness but no peritonism. Previously he had an appendicectomy some 50 years ago.

6.4.1 Diagnosis and management

This is the typical history of adhesive small bowel obstruction. Adhesive small bowel obstruction is uncommon in patients without previous surgery but 2–20% of patients who have had previous surgery will develop adhesive problems depending on the type of surgery. Previous surgery to the mid or lower abdomen is more likely to result in the band adhesions that are a major cause of subsequent small bowel obstruction (Parker *et al.* 2001). Onset is usually acute and results in referral to hospital. The diagnosis is made by the history of colicky central abdominal pain, presence of abdominal distension, plain abdominal films showing dilated small bowel, and by CT scan if necessary. An initial trial of conservative management, with nasogastric aspiration and intravenous fluid resuscitation is usual, but failure to resolve within 24 hours or associated signs of possible bowel infarction such as abdominal tenderness, raised white cell count, or CRP would mandate laparotomy.

6.4.2 Differential diagnosis

In the patient with a similar history an alternative cause of small bowel obstruction could be strangulation of a femoral, inguinal, or para-umbilical, or other hernia which would be detected on clinical examination. Because the caecum, ascending and transverse colon are also midgut structures, the colicky pain resulting from an obstructing right-sided colon carcinoma would present in a similar way with central colicky abdominal pain. In this instance the history is likely to be longer and associated with a change of bowel habit. Diagnosis in this case would be made by barium enema or colonoscopy and, in case of acute presentation, by plain abdominal films and CT. Iron deficiency anaemia is also a common presentation of a right-sided colonic malignancy, usually without abdominal pain. Iron deficiency anaemia in older people should be investigated for a possible large bowel cancer.

Although uncommon, small bowel ischaemia due to atherosclerosis and narrowing of the superior mesenteric artery can also present with central abdominal pain. In these circumstances there are more likely associated features of weight loss, malabsorption, and characteristic pain after meals. Because of the development of collateral circulation this is uncommon unless all the three arteries to the gut are involved—the coeliac axis, superior mesenteric, and inferior mesenteric arteries. Diagnosis can be made by either CT or MRI angiography. In contrast, acute mesenteric ischaemia caused by mesenteric artery embolus presents in a more acute manner with catastrophic generalized abdominal pain and shock and usually progresses rapidly to become fatal.

6.5 Lower abdominal pain

Box 6.3 Case study 3

Mrs White is an 83-year-old who presents to her general practitioner with a four-month history of colicky lower abdominal pain. This is intermittent but settles after she has opened her bowels. Her bowel habit has changed in that she used to open her bowels once daily but now she can go two to three times per day. Her stools are less formed than previously and there has been no blood in the stool. Both abdominal and rectal examinations are normal.

6.5.1 Diagnosis and management

This is the classical history of a left-sided colonic carcinoma. Any patient with such a history should obviously be investigated early by either flexible sigmoidoscopy, barium enema, or colonoscopy depending on the presentation (NICE guidelines, 2004b). Treatment is by resection following staging and results of surgery are comparable to younger patients, again dependent on co-morbidity.

6.5.2 Differential diagnosis

If the above patient does not present with the initial change in bowel habit then progression to a large bowel obstruction, is not uncommon. In this instance there is often the above history and then a few days onset of abdominal distension with colicky pain and absolute constipation. In this situation surgery has a higher morbidity and mortality and is less likely to result in a primary anastomosis and more likely a stoma as primary anastomosis is more difficult in the emergency setting.

Recurrent inflammation and severe diverticular disease can also result in a change in bowel habit and even colonic obstruction, although less commonly than malignancy. The typical history of diverticular disease is that of alternating constipation and diarrhoea. Episodes of diverticulitis are common in older patients as diverticular disease is extremely common. In this instance localized tenderness in the left iliac fossa is the most common presentation in association with pyrexia and raised white cell count. This will usually respond to antibiotic treatment although the development of a para-colonic abscess would make resolution unlikely and further intervention would be required.

6.6 Peritonitis

Box 6.4 Case study 4

Mr Smith is a 79-year-old who collapses with generalized abdominal and back pain. He is admitted to the accident and emergency department where he is observed to be pale and sweaty. He has a tachycardia and is hypotensive with a blood pressure of 70/40. Abdominal examination reveals generalized tenderness with peritonism and a pulsatile central abdominal mass.

6.6.1 Diagnosis and management

The diagnosis here is a ruptured aortic aneurysm and early intervention and repair is essential to prevent death. Ruptured aortic aneurysm in older patients results in a very high mortality and morbidity, as there is always associated co-morbidity secondary to arteriosclerosis.

6.6.2 Differential diagnosis

In the absence of a palpable abdominal mass there are numerous possible diagnoses as any intra-abdominal pathology resulting in peritonitis could present in a similar manner (Box 6.5). Diagnoses to be considered here include: perforated gastric or duodenal ulceration; pancreatitis; acute small bowel infarction, often in association with atrial fibrillation and an embolic mesenteric vascular occlusion; perforated appendicitis; purulent or faecal peritonitis due to diverticulitis; stercoral perforation or perforation secondary to colonic obstruction. After initial resuscitation, further investigation with plain abdominal films, CT scan or further clinical evaluation would result in a decision regarding the possibility of surgical intervention.

Box 6.5 Causes of generalized peritonitis

- Perforated gastric ulceration
- Perforated duodenal ulceration
- Pancreatitis
- Small bowel infarction in association with acute mesenteric ischaemia
- Small bowel infarction in association with closed loop obstruction
- Perforated appendicitis
- Perforated caecum in association with distal colonic obstruction
- Purulent peritonitis in association with perforated diverticulitis
- Faecal peritonitis in association with perforated diverticulitis
- Stercoral colonic perforation

6.7 Conclusions

The causes of abdominal pain are numerous and can lead to both routine and emergency consultations. Diagnosis is based on the site, onset, and character of the abdominal pain together with the presence or absence of abdominal signs on examination and the knowledge of the likelihood of different intra-abdominal pathologies. Management is based on investigations employed to establish a diagnosis followed by specific treatment of the underlying cause. Whether the treatment is conservative or active depends on knowledge of the natural history of the underlying problem.

References

Bingener J, Richards ML, Schwesinger WH, *et al.* (2003). Laparoscopic cholecystectomy for elderly patients: gold standard for golden years? *Arch Surg*, **138**(5), 531–5.

Blustein PK, Beck PL, Meddings JB, *et al.* (1998). The utility of endoscopy in the management of patients with gastroesophageal reflux symptoms. *Am J Gastroenterol*, **93**, 2508–12.

Halldestam I, Enell EL, Kullman E, *et al.* (2004). Development of symptoms and complications in individuals with asymptomatic gallstones. *Br J Surg*, **91**(6), 734–8.

Hilliard AA, Weinberger SE, Tierney LM Jr, *et al.* (2004). Clinical problem-solving. Occam's razor versus Saint's Triad. *N Engl J Med*, **350**(6), 599–603.

National Institute for Clinical Excellence (2004a). *Dyspepsia: managing dyspepsia in adults in primary care.* NICE, London. www.nice.org.uk/pdf/CG017fullguideline.pdf

National Institute for Clinical Excellence. (2004b). *Improving outcomes in colorectal cancer*. NICE, London. www.nice.org.uk/pdf/CSGCCfull guidance.pdf

Parker MJ, Ellis H, Moran BJ, *et al.* (2001). Postoperative adhesions: ten-year follow-up of 12,584 patients undergoing lower abdominal surgery. *Dis Colon Rectum*, **44**(6), 822–29.

Pring CM, Skelding-Millar L, Goodall RJ (2005). Expectant treatment or cholecystectomy after endoscopic retrograde cholangiopancreatography for choledocholithiasis in patients over 80 years old? *Surg Endosc*, **19**(3), 357–60.

Chapter 7

Medication for pain

Peter Crome

Key points

- Older people are the group that take the most prescribed and over-the-counter drugs and are at greatest risk of adverse drug reactions. However, they are also the group with the least evidence base to guide effective treatment.
- Frail older people are particularly vulnerable to the adverse effects of drugs.
- As a rule, potent analgesics should be started in lower doses.
- Vigilance is required to detect adverse drug reactions which may be atypical in presentation.
- Fear of causing adverse effects should not be an excuse for under treatment of pain.

7.1 Introduction

The effective and safe use of drugs to treat pain in older people poses special challenges. In general terms these challenges are little different to those posed by prescribing other classes of drugs—increased risk of adverse events, alterations in pharmacokinetics and pharmacodynamics, the poor evidence base to guide prescribing, and the enormous heterogeneity that exists within this age group. However, since many analgesic drugs have a narrow therapeutic index, their overuse may not only lead to intoxication, but also may pose a risk of addiction (Chapter 8). All of the above factors, which interact with the effects of co-morbidity and concomitant drug administration (both prescribed and over-the-counter), need to be taken into account when determining how drugs are to be prescribed and how drug treatment is to be monitored. This chapter presents a general overview of the clinical pharmacology of old age as well as describing key points relating to the use of the most commonly prescribed analgesic and adjuvant drugs.

7.2 Multiple prescribing

Older people are prescribed more drugs than those who are younger and absolute numbers of prescriptions in this age group are increasing (Information Centre for Health and Social Care, 2005). It is not uncommon for older people to be taking eight or more different drugs (Nielsen *et al.* 1981). The reason for this increase in prescribing is related to the higher prevalence of diseases in later life many of which are associated with pain—osteoarthritis, osteoporosis, and cancer being obvious examples. In addition, new classes of drugs continue to be developed including some for conditions which previously had no specific treatment e.g. cholinesterase-inhibitors for Alzheimer's disease. Further factors are policies which seek to ensure that all patients who might benefit from drugs receive them. National Service Frameworks (Department of Health, 2001), NICE (National Institute for Clinical Excellence, 2001) and other guidelines exemplify this issue. These trends are likely to continue.

7.3 Adverse drug events

Age and number of drugs taken are not surprisingly predictors of the risk of adverse drug events (Routledge *et al.* 2004). The potential for drug interactions increases exponentially with increasing numbers of prescribed drugs. Most adverse events are due to an excess pharmacological effect although some are due to unexpected idiosyncratic reactions. Adverse events continue to result in a significant number of hospital admissions and occupied bed days (Wiffen *et al.* 2002) despite a wider knowledge of the risks of drugs in older people. The consequences may be greater than in younger people. Thus a bleeding peptic ulcer caused by a non-steroidal anti-inflammatory drug is more likely to prove fatal and a fall caused by the sedative effect of an opioid is more likely to cause a osteoporotic fracture. Adverse events may also present in a non-specific fashion. Tiredness, anorexia, and reduced mobility are common in older people and may be drug related. There should be a high suspicion of adverse drug events.

7.4 Altered pharmacokinetics

The way in which drugs move through the body is described as pharmacokinetics. In normal ageing, changes in body composition, and in liver and kidney size and function, may alter this. In those with ill health or frailty, pharmacokinetic changes may be even more marked. As a result both the half-life of a drug may be prolonged and its clearance reduced. The effects of these alterations are shown in Table 7.1. The most predictable effects occur with drugs that are eliminated unchanged by the kidneys. With those drugs which are metabolized in the liver the effect is more variable. The balance between giving an ineffective dose, an effective dose, and a dose that produces side-effects is one of the major challenges in prescribing for older people.

7.5 Altered pharmacodynamics

The term pharmacodynamics is used to describe the way in which the drug affects the body and many drugs have a greater effect (both therapeutic and adverse) per unit dose in older people. This increased sensitivity may be due to changes at the cellular, tissue, or organ level, or to alterations in the body's homeostatic mechanisms and will require dose reduction. It should be noted that there are a small number of drugs to which older people are relatively resistant. For example, beta-receptor agonists and antagonist have to be given in larger doses to produce the same effect.

7.6 Concordance and health beliefs

The term concordance is now preferred to compliance and describes the way in which patients use drugs. It implies a greater partnership between the prescriber and the patient. Confusion, inability to open bottles or other containers, poor eyesight, and misunderstandings may all result in patients not taking the drug as the prescriber had intended. The key to successful concordance is an exploration of patients' beliefs about their illness and the drugs which are prescribed. Many patients believe that analgesic drugs will lead to addiction and dependence and that they will in some way oppose natural body healing or hasten decline. Although one may not be able to change patients' erroneous views, understanding of them will improve prescriber-patient relationships.

Table 7.1 Consequences of pharmacokinetic changes on drug prescription

Pharmacokinetic change	Effect
Increased half-life	Longer to reach steady-state Longer for plasma concentrations to fall
Reduced clearance	Higher plasma concentrations and greater therapeutic effect Greater risk of dose-related adverse events

7.7 Inappropriate drugs and drug combinations

The high frequency of adverse drug events in older people has led to the development of lists of drugs which are considered to be of limited value and excessive risk. They can apply to all older people, to those with specific conditions or to specific combinations with other drugs. The most widely used are the Beers criteria, last updated in 2003 (Fick *et al.* 2003). Included in his list are indomethacin and amitriptyline. This list may be a useful method for auditing practice and requires regular review as new evidence emerges.

7.8 The evidence-deficit

Perhaps the biggest issue is that of the lack of an adequate evidence base for the rational use of drugs in people over the age of eighty. Older people are not recruited into clinical trials in sufficient numbers despite regulatory authority guidance indicating that this should happen (The International Conference on Harmonisation Harmonised Tripartite Guideline, 1994). This applies to both trials that compare drugs against placebo as well as to head-to-head comparisons between new and well established medications. This is perhaps of lesser importance in analgesic drugs which are given in the short-term for symptomatic relief but is of importance when drugs are given over a long time with the primary aim of preventing pain or disease progression. Getting the balance right between therapeutic nihilism and an over-optimistic view of a drug's worth is challenging. It is of course important to understand that lack of evidence of the efficacy of a drug is not the same as evidence of lack of efficacy of that agent.

7.9 Principles of drug choice: the stepped approach

The general principles for the treatment of pain in older people are no different than for those in younger patients. Non-pharmacological approaches and the local use of analgesics need to be considered. Age alone should never be a reason for non-referral to specialist pain and other services where consideration for alternative approaches may be given (surgery, nerve blocks etc). For a recent review of interventional approaches see Bernstein *et al.* (2005). However, for many, if not the majority of patients, analgesic drugs will be required and for the reasons stated above such treatment can be more problematic than in younger people. Diagnostic difficulties, fear of causing adverse effects, and concordance issues should never be an excuse for inadequate treatment and the evidence does suggest that older people are often under treated (Jones *et al.* 1996).

Drugs used for the treatment of pain are conventionally classified as analgesics (principally non-steroidal anti-inflammatory drugs and opioids) or adjuvants such as antidepressants and anti-epileptic agents.

Table 7.2 Classification of analgesic drugs (not comprehensive)

Non-opioid drugs	• Aspirin • Nefopam • Paracetamol
Selective cyclo-oxygenase 2 inhibitors	• Celecoxib • Etoricoxib • Lumiracoxib
Non-steroidal anti-inflammatory drugs (NSAIDs)	• Aceclofenac • Diclofenac • Diflusinal • Etodalac • Fenbufen • Fenoprofen • Flurbiprofen • Ibuprofen • Indometacin • Ketoprofen • Meloxicam • Nabumetone • Naproxen • Piroxicam • Sulindac • Tenoxicam • Tiaprofenic acid
Compound analgesics	• Aspirin + codeine • Paracetamol + codeine • Paracetamol + dihydrocodeine • Paracetamol + tramadol
Opioid drugs	• Buprenorphine** • Codeine • Diamorphine • Dihydrocodeine • Fentanyl** • Meptazinol • Methadone • Oxycodone • Tramadol*

* Not suitable for opioid dependent patients

** Available as patches

Analgesic drugs themselves are subdivided into the non-opioid analgesics, which include the non-steroidal anti-inflammatory drugs, and the opioids. As a broad generalization the non-opioid drugs are preferred for musculo-skeletal conditions (Chapters 4 and 5) whilst more potent opioids are used for visceral pain (Chapter 6). Table 7.2 lists analgesic drugs available in the United Kingdom.

For chronic or persistent pain, whether due to benign or to malignant conditions, a stepped approach is recommended. The most widely known in the WHO ladder for malignant pain (see Chapter 13). The actual drugs recommended at each stage vary from guideline to guideline. As an example, a new guideline for arthritic pain recommends low dose buprenorphine patches as an alternative at Stage II (Figure 7.1 modified from Serpell *et al.* 2006). Optimal treatment may require the use of combinations of drugs such as the addition of an anti-inflammatory drug or an adjuvant drug with an opioid. The step approach has been adapted for many of the other symptoms such as cough and vomiting which cause distress in terminally ill patients (Twycross *et al.* 2002).

Figure 7.1 Algorithm for the management of pain in patients with osteoarthritis

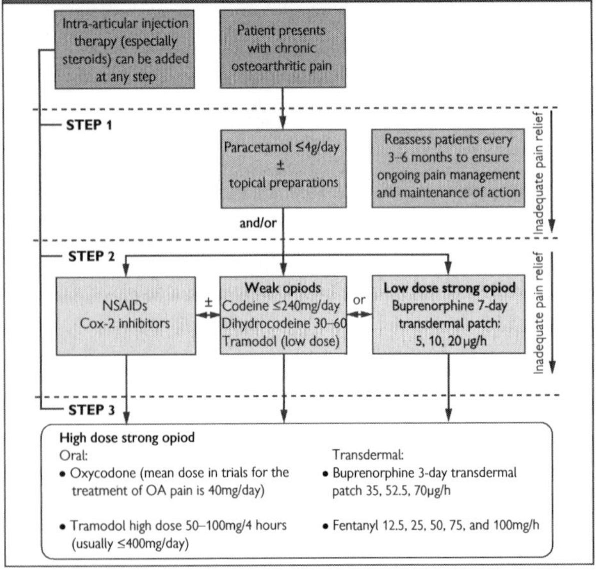

For acute pain the choice will depend on diagnosis and judgement of severity. Thus conditions which are clearly associated with severe pain (e.g. fracture femur, myocardial infarction) demand that a potent drug such as morphine is prescribed. It is not appropriate to give a mild analgesic and wait to see whether it is effective. However, in older people diagnosis may be difficult, particularly in those with cognitive impairment or co-morbidity. Uncertainty demands frequent review both of the diagnosis and of the efficacy of pain relief.

There are a large number of analgesic drugs available and knowledge about their therapeutic and adverse effects is continually emerging.

7.10 Choice of dose frequency and route

For localized pain, local drug treatment may be appropriate. For those who are unconscious or who have swallowing difficulties, drugs may be given by injection or suppository. However, for most the oral route is preferred. The frequency of dosing will depend on the pharmacokinetics of the drug and the clinical course of the disease. For malignant pain the mantra 'by the clock', 'by the mouth', and 'by the ladder' together with individual and regular review is required.

7.11 Over-the-counter drugs available for mild pain

7.11.1 Paracetamol (acetaminophen)

This is the drug of choice, being virtually devoid of side effects at normal therapeutic doses. The major potential disadvantage is that it is toxic when taken in overdose causing hepatic and renal failure although the effects can be reduced if the antidote acetylcysteine is given in time. Reductions in drug clearance have been found in frail older people but dosage reduction is probably not needed.

7.11.2 Aspirin

Aspirin has anti-platelet aggregation, antipyretic, and anti-inflammatory actions as well as analgesic properties. It is widely used for the prevention of cardiovascular and cerebrovascular disease.

Box 7.1

Unless prescribers are confident that they have up-to-date knowledge about a particular drug or combination of drugs then they should consult current reference works such as the *British National Formulary* (2006). This is also available on the internet (www.bnf.org.uk).

The main drawback to its use is that it causes gastrointestinal irritation and erosion leading to discomfort and blood loss which may be severe. In addition a small number of patients display allergic reactions. Its use as an analgesic is best reserved for those who are taking the drug already without side effects and those patients who are intolerant to paracetamol.

7.11.3 **Ibuprofen**

This drug acts by inhibiting the enzyme cyclo-oxygenase and reducing the production of pain and inflammation-producing substances. In low, over-the-counter doses, it is well tolerated but in higher doses it can cause gastrointestinal haemorrhage and perforation. It is principally for this reason that paracetamol is preferred as the analgesic of choice in older people.

7.11.4 **Combination analgesics**

There are a number of over-the-counter formulations that combine paracetamol and low-dose or low potency opioid drugs. The evidence that combination tablets are more effective is not great.

7.12 Prescription Drugs

7.12.1 **Non-opioid drugs**

There are a large number of non-steroidal anti-inflammatory drugs in addition to ibuprofen which has previously been mentioned (see Table 7.2). They have both analgesic and anti-inflammatory properties and are therefore particularly appropriate for arthritic conditions (see Chapter 5). The principal problem with their use is gastrointestinal haemorrhage and the presence of, or history of, peptic ulcer is a contra-indication. For high risk patients gastro-protective agents may be co-prescribed. In addition they cause fluid retention and may aggravate both cardiac and renal failure. Their use in patients with either of these co-morbidities, which are themselves age-related, requires close monitoring.

COX-2 inhibitors have less effect on gastrointestinal mucosa and for this reason have been advocated as first-line drugs for older people. However, they may have an adverse effect on cardiac and renal function and in addition are pro-thrombogenic, their use having been associated with an increased risk of stroke and myocardial infarction. One drug of this class (rofecoxib) has been withdrawn for this reason. Established vascular disease of any type is a contra-indication to their use whilst caution is needed in the presence of vascular risk factors. There is also a possibility that other non-steroidal anti-inflammatory drugs may also be thrombogenic but this is not clearly established. The basic advice for the use of all non-steroidal anti-inflammatory drugs including COX-2 is to use the lowest dose for the shortest time (Commission on Human Medicines and Medicines and Healthcare Products Regulatory Agency 2006).

7.12.2 **Opioid analgesics**

These are most potent analgesic drugs. Those in common use such as morphine and codeine exert their effects through central μ_1 receptor. Other drugs such as buprenorphine and tramadol have more complicated pharmacological actions. These drugs have a large number of side effects some of which may be difficult to recognize in older people (Table 7.3). A high degree of suspicion that symptoms may be due to adverse effects is required and any deterioration in a patient's condition should not automatically be assumed to be due to progression of disease. The risks of the patient developing addiction to the drugs are small but real. Extra care is needed when treating older patients with alcoholism, psychiatric co-morbidity, or personality disorders.

Morphine is the most commonly used opioid and has the advantage of being available in several formulations including oral liquid and slow-release preparations as well as solutions for subcutaneous

Table 7.3 Side effects of opioid drugs

Central nervous system	• Tolerance • Drowsiness* • Ataxia • Coma • Falls • Seizures • Movement disorders • Nausea and vomiting* • Pupillary constriction • Confusion* • Hallucinations*
Cardiovascular system	• Hypotension • Vagal bradycardia
Respiratory system	• Respiratory depression • Hypoxia and hypercapnoea • Cough suppression
Gastrointestinal system	• Dry mouth • Increased oesophageal reflux • Delayed gastric emptying and gastro-intestinal motility • Constipation* • Abdominal pain
Urinary system	• Urinary retention

* Common

infusions. The overall effect of pharmacokinetic changes is that smaller doses are needed in older people for any given effect. The usual starting dose for morphine when used for chronic pain is 5–10mg every four hours with half that dose being used in the frail with additional doses given for breakthrough pain. Patients then should be switched to a twice-daily sustained release preparation with additional doses of one-sixth the total daily dose being used for breakthrough pain. If increasing the dose by 30–50% does not produce a response, consider muscle spasm or neuropathic pain. Conversion charts exist for giving equivalent analgesic doses of other opioids when morphine appears not to be effective.

If opiods are used long-term, consideration should be given to the addition of a laxative (senna and lactulose or codanthramer). If nausea and vomiting becomes a problem metoclopramide or haloperidol may be needed.

For patients with swallowing disorders or in whom concordance is a problem, the use of a patch preparation should be considered. Both buprenorphine and fentanyl are available in high dose whilst the former is also available in lower doses suitable for chronic non-malignant pain. Opioids may also be given by syringe drivers for patients who also have persistent nausea and vomiting, fluctuating consciousness, or malabsorption.

7.12.3 **Combination analgesics**

Coproxamol (the prescription-only combination of paracetamol and dextropropoxyphene) has been a widely used drug. Unfortunately the drug is highly toxic when taken in overdose, causing early cardio-respiratory depression and arrest especially when alcohol is also taken. Patients who recover from this early toxicity have been known to go on and develop paracetamol-induced liver failure. It is now being withdrawn in the United Kingdom. Codeine combinations are generally regarded as the step-up combination of choice. Constipation is a common problem and codeine can produce all the adverse effects of morphine if given in high doses.

7.12.4 **Adjuvant drugs**

Adjuvant drugs are used principally for neuropathic pains. Commonly used drugs include antidepressants (both tricyclic and SSRI) and anti-epileptic drugs including gabapentin, valproate, and carbamazepine. Tricyclic antidepressants (amitripyline is used most commonly) should be used cautiously because of their anti-cholinergic effects and in doses lower than usually employed for the treatment of depression (e.g. amitriptyline 10–25mg at night). The risk of cardiac toxicity has probably been overstated in the past but SSRIs are preferred in older patients with active heart disease. Capsaicin (the active component of chili powder) may be used locally taking the usual precautions not to get in the eye.

7.13 Specialist pain services

Specialist pain services are now provided in both hospitals and the community although access to them for older people may still be a problem. Services for palliative or terminal care may be separately provided from those for more chronic conditions. Government policies clearly state that older people should not be denied access to such services on account of age. It is important that any professional obstruction to access is removed.

7.14 Conclusions: improving prescribing

Optimal prescribing for the treatment and prevention of pain in older people is as dependent on knowledge derived from the patient as knowledge derived from the medical or pharmacological literature. Diagnosis, patient expectations, experiences, and beliefs should all be explored and the role of drugs should be placed alongside other treatment modalities.

When several different drugs are being taken, there should be a thorough review of what drugs are really necessary and those which are of marginal benefit may be discontinued. This is of more relevance to those with a short life expectancy. Drugs with short durations of actions need to be administered frequently and in anticipation of events that might aggravate pain. Regular review is essential and there should be a low threshold for altering dose and drug if effectiveness diminishes or side effects are suspected.

Prescribers need to know about the drugs they prescribe both to inform their practice and to inform patients. Generally speaking it is better to know more about a restricted range of drugs. For many drugs prescribed for older people the motto 'start low and go slow' is appropriate. However, in the case of analgesia it should not be so slow and so low that the patient gets no or little pain relief.

References

Bernstein C, Lateef B and Fine P (2005). Interventional pain management procedures in older patients. In Gibson SJ and Weiner DK (eds). *Pain in Older People*. IASP Press, Seattle.

British National Formulary: BNF51 (2006). BMJ Publishing Group London and RPS Publishing, London. (www.bnf.org).

Commission on Human Medicines and Medicines and Healthcare Products Regulatory Agency (2006). *Current Problems in Pharmacovigilance* **31**, 7.

Department of Health (2001). *Medicines and older people—Implementing medicines-related aspects of the NSF for older people.* DoH, London.

Information Centre for health and social care (2005). *Prescriptions dispensed in the community: Statistics for 1994 to 2004—England.* DH, London.

Crome P and Ford G (eds) (2000). *Drugs and the Older Population.* Imperial College Press, London.

Fick DM, Cooper JW, Wade WE *et al.* (2003). Updating the Beers criteria for potentially inappropriate medication use in older adults: results of a US consensus panel of experts. *Arch. Intern. Med.* **163**, 2716–24.

Jones JS, Johnson K, and McNinch M (1996). Age as a risk factor for inadequate emergency department analgesia. *American Journal of Emergency Medicine*, **14**, 157–60.

National Institute for Clinical Excellence (2001). *Guidance on the use of donepezil, rivastigmine and galantamine for the treatment of Alzheimer's Disease.* NICE, London.

Nielsen IK, Osterlind AW, Christiansen LV, *et al.* (1981). 'Drug consumption and age in a department of internal medicine'. *Dan Med Bull*, **28**, (2), 71–3.

Routledge PA, O'Mahony MS, and Woodhouse KW (2004). 'Adverse drug reactions in elderly patients'. *British Journal of Clinical Pharmacology*, **57**, (2), 121–6.

Serpell M, Conaghan P, Crome P, *et al.* (2006). Primary care treatment and management of chronic osteoarthritic pain. *e-Guidelines*, **28**, 353–7.

The International Conference on Harmonisation Harmonised Tripartite Guideline (1994). Studies in support of special populations: geriatrics. London.

Twycross R, Wilcock A, Charlesworth S, *et al.* (2002). Palliative Care Formulary. Radcliffe Medical Press, Oxford.

Wiffen P, Gill M, Edwards J, *et al.* (2002). Adverse drug reactions in hospital patients: a systematic review of the prospective and retrospective studies. *Bandolier Extra*, **June**, 1–14.

Further reading

AGS Panel on Persistent Pain in Older People (2002). The management of persistent pain in older persons. *JAGS*, **50**, S205–S224.

Gibson SJ and Weiner DK (eds). *Pain in Older People.* IASP Press, Seattle.

Chapter 8

Pain and addiction

Ilana Crome

Key points

- Considerable numbers of older people are misusing tobacco, alcohol, illicit drugs, over-the-counter medications, and prescribed medications.
- Physicians lack confidence in the assessment and treatment of these conditions.
- Substance problems are unrecognized and under-treated in older people.
- Addictive behaviour needs to be taken seriously in older people presenting with pain.
- Thorough assessment of pain should take account of the physical, psychological, and social components of the background.
- Assessment should include a high index of suspicion about current or potential addictive behaviour, development of substance problems or dependence (addiction).
- There are specific diagnostic criteria for the differentiation of harmful substance use and dependence (addiction).
- Treatment choices depend on the ability to make the distinction between harmful use and dependence.
- Treatment interventions for addiction problems are effective.
- Treatment of addiction problems may be even more effective in older people than in younger age groups.
- Treatment of the addict in pain is best undertaken by a multidisciplinary team.

8.1 Introduction

Patients with chronic pain who are refractory to treatment are a challenge to practitioners. Substance problems are an unrecognized issue, which physicians are ill-prepared to evaluate. This chapter provides the perspective of an addiction specialist, as it considers use, misuse, and dependence (addiction) on substances and the mechanisms of relationships to pain, as well as assessment and treatment of addiction. Undertreatment of pain may lead to addiction in patients with a history of substance misuse. The impact on service provision and policy will be discussed.

8.2 What is a drug?

The term 'drug' will be used to cover tobacco and alcohol, illicit substances, central nervous system depressants (opiates and opioids, e.g. heroin and methadone), and stimulants (cocaine, crack, amphetamines, and ecstasy). It includes 'street' use and use of prescription drugs (such as benzodiazepines) in a manner that is **not** indicated or intended by a medical practitioner and using over-the-counter preparations such as codeine-based products, e.g. cough medicines, decongestants, other than in accordance with instructions. Older people may use a combination of these (so-called 'polypharmacy' or 'polydrug' 'misuse' or 'dependence') in an effort to control pain, which may be associated with physical or psychological comorbidity. The role of the practitioner is to attempt to separate out whether the medication or substance use is in addition to treatment being taken for pain control (Crome & Bloor in press; Crome & Ghodse in press).

8.3 Terminology *is* important: what exactly is addiction?

The terms 'substance' and 'drug' will be used interchangeably. In order to reach a 'diagnosis', the two systems that have emerged are the International Classification of Diseases (ICD-10) (World Health Organization, 1992) and the American Psychiatric Association's Diagnostic and Statistical Manual (DSM IV) (1994). The criteria required to reach a diagnosis of either harmful use or dependent use are to be found in Boxes 8.1 and 8.2. These systems have similarities, but they are not identical. *The* most important issue is to be able to determine, with regard to a wide range of substances, whether patients are engaging in harmful use or are dependent. This differentiation is critical in terms of decisions around the selection of appropriate treatment interventions (with regards to type and intensity) and suitability of settings.

Box 8.1 Criteria for substance abuse (DSM IV) and harmful use (ICD 10)

DSM IV (APA, 1994) describes substance abuse as follows:

A maladaptive pattern of substance use leading to clinically significant impairment or distress, as manifested by one (or more) of the following occurring within a 12-month period:

- Recurrent substance use resulting in a failure to fulfil major role obligations at work, school, or home.
- Recurrent substance-abuse-related legal problems.
- Continued substance abuse despite having persistent or recurrent social or interpersonal problems caused or exacerbated by the effects of the substance.
- Has never met the criteria for substance dependence for this class of substance.

ICD 10 (WHO, 1992) has a far simpler definition i.e.

- A pattern of psychoactive substance use that is causing damage to health; the damage may be to physical or mental health.

In essence the two classificatory systems note that use of substances can be damaging and harmful in physical, psychological, and social domains without meeting the criteria for the addiction or dependence syndrome.

Box 8.2 Criteria for dependence syndrome in DSM IV and ICD 10

Both DSM IV and ICD 10 are fundamentally very similar and propose a diagnosis of dependence on a substance should be made if three (or more) of the following have been experienced or exhibited during the previous year:

- Tolerance: this develops when there is either need for markedly increased amount of substance to achieve intoxication or desired effect, or markedly diminished effect with continued use of the same amount of the substance.
- Withdrawal state: this is evidenced by the characteristic withdrawal syndrome for the substance when it is not available, or if the same (or closely related) substance is taken to relieve or avoid withdrawal symptom.
- Control: difficulties in controlling substance-taking behaviour in terms of its onset, termination, or levels of use. Thus, the substance is often taken in larger amounts over a longer period of time than was intended and there is a persistent desire or repeated unsuccessful efforts to cut down or control substance use.
- Persistent use: persistence in using substances despite clear evidence of overly harmful consequences (physical or mental).
- Neglect of obligations: progressive neglect of alternative pleasures or interests because of psychoactive substance use and increased amount of time necessary to obtain or take the substance or to recover from its effect.
- Only ICD 10 uses the criterion of compulsion or a strong desire to take the substance.

8.4 Epidemiology

One in ten older people are receiving a drug that is potentially inappropriate (Gottlieb, 2004). Older people receive most of the prescriptions in the UK and are being dispensed multiple medications (McGrath *et al.* 2005). Over-the-counter availability (or obtaining medicines other than through legitimate channels) makes multiple analgesic drug use a particular problem (Chrischilles *et al.* 1990). Although 'drug misuse' is often perceived as the domain of young people, increasingly those dependent on opiates and other illicit drugs in young adulthood do survive into old age (Lynskey *et al.* 2003; Office for National Statistics, 2001). A national study of psychiatric morbidity showed decreases in use of any illicit drugs from age 55 to 69 but an increase among those in the 70–74 age group (Coulthard *et al.* 2002) (see Table 8.1).

Almost 10% of those in the 55–59 age group who had ever taken drugs had experienced an overdose, as had 5% of those in the over 60 age group. Although the prevalence of smoking in the over 60s is

Table 8.1 Use of any illicit drug/1000 population by age group

Age	55–59	60–64	65–69	70–74
Lifetime use	84/1000	65/1000	24/1000	34/1000
Last year use	19/1000	10/1000	6/1000	11/1000
Last month use	7/1000	7/1000	2/1000	2/1000

Adapted from Coulthard *et al.* (2002).

Box 8.3 Demographic factors influencing substance misuse in older people

- Alcohol use decreases with increasing age.
- 61% in the 65–69 age group had a drink in the last week compared to 44% in the 85–89 age group (ONS, 2001).
- Psychotropic drug misuse is greater in women than in men.
- Older women drink less, they smoke less and use less illicit drugs than other age-gender groups (Kelly, 2003; Graham *et al.* 1995).
- 26% of elderly men had drunk on 5 or more days prior to interview, compared to 15% of women (Office for National Statistics, 2001).

decreasing, about 20% of 60–64-year-olds, 15% of 65–69-year-olds, and 10% of 70–74-year-olds still smoke. Information on the over 80s is scarce, although this is the largest growing group of older people.

8.5 Pain and addiction

Addictive behaviour needs to be taken seriously in older people presenting with pain. About 12% of patients presenting at an adult pain clinic have a substance disorder (Kouyanou *et al.* 1997). Older problem drinkers report more severe pain, more disruption of daily activities due to pain and more frequent use of alcohol to manage pain than older non-problem drinkers (Brennan *et al.* 2005). The association with pain and self-harm has been demonstrated (Theodoulou *et al.* 2005). Pain can interfere with treatment: in a study of a substance misuse residential unit for veterans, it was found that those with back pain were less likely to complete treatment than those without back pain (Stack *et al.* 2000). Therefore, detection is important for appropriate treatment.

8.6 Assessment of substance use disorder

There are three elements to the comprehensive assessment: pain, substance misuse, and psychosocial background. The practitioner must assess why the patient is presenting for treatment; the features of the pain (time course, intensity, location, quality, exacerbating factors); the use (compliant or otherwise) of prescription drugs and over-the-counter medication; and alcohol, nicotine, and illicit drug use, misuse, and dependence. The assessment of quantity and frequency of use, route (oral, smoking, intravenous), combinations and potential interactions is important. A history of substance misuse in the past, treatment and treatment outcome, and history of self harm should be elicited. The family history as well as psychiatric, medical, and social (including forensic) problems should be probed. How this information fits in with a possible diagnosis of substance misuse or dependence should be considered. Confirmation should be sought from a clinical physical and mental state examination, especially evidence of withdrawal or intoxication for specific drugs, and including evidence of current suicidal ideation. Evidence of the relationship of pain to the effects of substance use, i.e. neurological, hepatic, renal, respiratory or cardiac difficulties, injecting behaviour (abscesses, cellulitis or septicaemia), needs specific analysis. Biochemical, haematological investigations and urinalysis should be undertaken.

The key judgement to be made relates to the nature and extent of the pain, to whether the patient appears to be displaying the behavioural characteristics of 'drug seeking' and to whether this is related to inadequate prescribing for the pain, or not. The behaviours that have been identified include selling, forging, losing, borrowing and stealing prescriptions, non-compliance, unsanctioned dose escalation, requests for renewal or medical before the due date, and seeking prescriptions from a variety of medical practitioners and sources (Chabal *et al.* 1997; Jaffe, 1992; Portenoy & Payne, 1997; Savage, 1996). Patients may focus on medication during consultations, complain about the need for more drugs, be unwilling to reduce medication, and refuse other pharmacological or non-pharmacological treatments. However, some patients may be on sub-optimal doses required to control pain and, though they might exhibit such behaviours for a time, once their medication is stabilized, this situation (so-called 'pseudo-addiction') reverses.

Screening instruments can be useful for the identification of substance use and pain. There are a number of assessment tools for screening for substance use and misuse (Crome & Bloor, 2006), (see Tables 8.2 and 8.3). Several instruments have been developed for screening potential opiate medication misuse in chronic pain patients (Adams *et al.* 2004; Chabal *et al.* 1997; Compton *et al.* 1998; Friedman *et al.* 2003). Adams *et al.* (2004) have reported on the Pain Medication Questionnaire (PMQ), which assesses potential opioid misuse in chronic pain patients. A history of substance misuse, higher levels of psychological distress and poorer functioning were predictive of opioid misuse. Michna *et al.* (2004) reported that a family history of substance misuse and a history of legal problems and drug and alcohol misuse were likely to manifest more 'aberrant drug related behaviours'. Friedman *et al.* (2003), using the Screening Tool for Addiction Risk (STAR), suggests that a prior history of substance misuse treatment and nicotine dependence might distinguish patients with pain and substance misuse from those with pain only. Schieffer *et al.* (2005) have demonstrated that a history of substance misuse is associated with increased opiate misuse independent of differences in reported opiate effectiveness.

8.7 Mechanisms of relationships between pain and substance use, misuse, and dependence

The comorbidity of pain and substance misuse and dependence may present with many different permutations (Crome, 1999). Substance use—even one dose—may lead to a traumatic event, such as a fall, road traffic accident, or head injury as a result of intoxication. Harmful use and dependence on drugs may produce painful conditions, e.g. abscesses, cellulitis, chest pain (see Boxes 8.4 and 8.5), as may withdrawal from a substance, for instance opiate withdrawal. Pain may drive a substance use disorder, i.e. may lead to increased substance use, and pain may be associated with mental health problems (e.g. depression, post traumatic stress disorder, anxiety).

Table 8.2 Useful substance misuse screening questionnaires*

Instrument	Description
ARPS (Moore *et al.* 1999; Nguyen *et al.* 2001)	A 60-item self-administered questionnaire, which identifies 3 types of drinkers: 1) harmful drinkers, 2) hazardous drinkers and 3) abstainers and non-hazardous drinkers. A 32-item version, the ShARPS, is also available.
CAGE (Ewing, 1984; Mayfield *et al.* 1974)	General population questionnaire consisting of 4 items: 1) Have you ever felt you should **c**ut down on your drinking?; 2) Have people **a**nnoyed you by criticising your drinking; 3) Have you ever felt bad or **g**uilty about your drinking; 4) Have you ever had a drink first thing in the morning to steady your nerves or to get rid of a hangover (**e**ye opener)? Useful in older people, but not validated.
MAST-G (Blow *et al.* 1992)	Specifically for use with older people. 24 items with yes/no answers, scoring 1 for yes and 0 for no. A score of 5 or above is indicative of an alcohol problem.

* Please note: there is a plethora of instruments available for assessing substance misuse. However, these are either aimed at older people or have been recommended for use with an older population in previous research.

Table 8.3 Screening instruments for addiction in chronic pain

Instrument	Description
Chabal *et al.* 1997	A five-item checklist, based on DSM-III-R criteria.
Prescription Drug Use Questionnaire (Compton *et al.* 1998)	A 40-item questionnaire. A score of 15 or more indicates substance use disorder and a score of 25 or more substance dependence.
PMQ (Adams *et al.* 2004)	A 26-item questionnaire.
STAR (Friedman *et al.* 2003)	A 14-item self-administered questionnaire.

Box 8.4 Physical comorbidity and alcohol

Trauma
- Head injury, fall, accident

Infection
- Neuropathy, e.g. vascular, trauma, viral and carcinoma.
- Thiamine deficiency
- Pellagra (niacin and protein deficiency) and scurvy (vitamin C deficiency) are less common (Cook *et al.* 1998).

Gastrointestinal disease
- Alcoholic fatty liver, hepatitis and cirrhosis (Baptista *et al.* 1981)
- Acute and chronic pancreatitis, gastritis and peptic ulcer

Carcinoma of the oral cavity, pharynx, hypopharynx, larynx, oesophagus, liver, colorectum, and the breast (Poschl & Seitz, 2004).

Cardiovascular disease
- Ischaemic stroke and coronary disease
- Haemorrhagic stroke,
- Cardiomyopathy,
- Hypertension
- Cardiac arrhythmias (Sesso, 2001)

Musculo skeletal disease
- Skeletal muscle myopathy
- Osteoporosis
- Fractures

Box 8.5 Physical comorbidity and drugs

The use of drugs by injection is a risk for infection with HIV but also carries with it a series of risks:
- Pneumonia
- Cellulitis
- Endocarditis
- Abscess (Stein, 1997).
- Injecting (including risk of HIV and Hepatitis B and C)
- Septicaemia

Cannabis:
Risk of lung cancer and cancers of the head and neck.

Amphetamines and cocaine:
- Chest pain and neurological problems such as seizure or stroke (Stein, 1997)
- Nasal septal perforation and damage to the nasal passages
- Hypertension, cardiac arrhythmias, stroke
- Hepatic and renal damage
- Pulmonary disease e.g. 'crack lung' and pulmonary oedema

The interrelationships between physical health (including pain), mental health and drug misuse are well documented. Apart from the direct effects of drugs on general health, there are indirect effects such as dietary neglect, impoverishment, trauma, bereavement and loss. Malnutrition, for instance, may emanate from drug-induced anorexia, malabsorption and economic deprivation. Liver dysfunction, e.g. HIV, hepatitis B and C, produces psychological as well as physical problems.

Psychiatric conditions, such as anxiety, depression, post-traumatic stress disorder, schizophrenia, delirium, and dementia may lead to, be a consequence of, or coincide with, substance misuse. Withdrawal from barbiturates and benzodiazepines leads to delirium, whereas head injuries and serious infections as a result of substance use disorder are associated with dementia.

Depression, dementia, delirium, and a heightened risk of suicide are probably the problems most commonly faced by clinicians. Of course, sometimes some of these conditions are associated with chronic pain and sleep disorders, which may make patients vulnerable and lead to them seeking relief from drugs. Sleep disorders such as insomnia (Beresford, 2000) may precipitate an increased alcohol intake and a consequent negative effect on sleep patterns. Pain may lead to functional decline, which may destabilize treatment for psychological and psychiatric conditions.

These complex interactions have implications in that not only does drug use interfere with emotional, cognitive, and social behaviour, but also the combination of disorders results in poorer treatment compliance and both short- and long-term outcome. The pharmacokinetic changes observed with increasing age may have an influence on propensity to dependence on a variety of substances and there is convincing evidence of age-related changes in drug metabolism for a variety of drugs including alcohol (Ozdemir *et al.* 1996).

8.8 Treatment effectiveness

Over the last ten years there have been steadily accumulating advances in the evaluation of treatment interventions for substance misuse (Gossop *et al.* 2003; UKATT Research Team, 2005). Overall findings indicate that outcome can be greatly improved.

8.8.1 Psychological approaches

Psychological therapies can be broadly described as behavioural, psychodynamic, self help, counselling, and brief interventions. Some of these approaches may also be of benefit for treatment of the painful condition. An assessment of controlled studies in substance misuse lists the 'top ten' interventions as brief interventions, motivational enhancement, acamprosate, naltrexone, social skills training, community reinforcement, behavioural contracting, behavioural marital therapy, case management, and self-monitoring (McLellan *et al.* 1999).

The use of brief physician advice for problem drinking has been shown to be of value. A minimal intervention at a primary care level results in a reduction in alcohol use in patients over 65 for a period of at least 24 months (Fleming *et al.* 1999; Mundt *et al.* 2005). The effect of brief interventions in patients over the age of 65 has been shown to be similar to the response of younger patients with alcohol problems (Gordon *et al.* 2003). Brief interventions have also been shown to reduce mortality by 23–36% in the population of problem drinkers (Cuijpers *et al.* 2004).

8.8.2 **Pharmacotherapy**

Pharmacological treatments are usually administered if patients are dependent on substances. There is a whole raft of interventions for alcohol, opiate, and nicotine dependence. Medications are used for withdrawal, detoxification, reduction and maintenance regimens, relapse prevention, and for the treatment of psychiatric disorder. As regards the treatment of alcohol withdrawal, it is clear that the elderly respond to interventions with the same degree of success as younger patients, and a recent review of the treatment of alcohol problems in the older patient emphasized the importance of providing adequate pharmacological and psychosocial interventions for this population (Whelan 2003). Naltrexone, acamprosate, and disulfiram should be used with extreme caution in older people and should only be prescribed by clinicians who are very experienced in using this medication, if at all. For opiate dependence, methadone and buprenorphine are commonly used, and for nicotine dependence, nicotine replacement or bupropion (though the latter should be used with caution in the older person) (for a detailed review see Lingford-Hughes *et al.* 2004).

In summary, though prescription of opiates as effective in chronic pain is well documented (Bouckoms *et al.* 1992; Jamison *et al.* 1994), there have also been concerns that the prescribing of long term opiates to patients with chronic non-cancer pain could lead to misuse and dependence. Despite a recent RCT study dispelling this notion (Cowan *et al.* 2005), some patients may misuse opiates and other medications and substances.

8.9 **The practicalities of treating an addict in pain**

This can be one of the most challenging clinical situations to manage (Littlejohn *et al.* 2004). This is partly because pain has a very strong subjective component. All members of the team treating the patient should be aware of the complexity of the situation, treat the patient with courtesy at all times, assess (and if needs be investigate) each symptom or complaint carefully, and reassure the patient that every effort is being made to help them. This can allay a great deal of disquiet on all sides.

There are two broad categories of populations:

- The addicted in pain and
- The pain patient with resulting addictive problems.

There are several important areas to consider.

The first issue is whether the patient is being undertreated for their painful condition, because many people, especially addicts, often are. Patients with substance dependence are usually very concerned that they will not be believed, tolerated, or adequately treated, and that their current medication will be reduced. It cannot be overemphasized how disabling and counterproductive the anxiety can be. The second issue is the nature of pain (e.g. acute or chronic, and whether is it non-malignant or malignant chronic pain), and how dysfunctional it is.

The third issue is that a judgement needs to be made regarding whether the degree of dysfunction is related to a psychological or psychiatric component. Assessment of current treatment, or the potential need for treatment, for the dependence, as well as for the physical and psychological problems, is required.

Consider a number of different scenarios:

- The patient who is currently stable on maintenance therapy for addiction e.g. methadone or buprenorphine.
- The patient who is unstable on maintenance therapy.
- The patient who had a history of addiction problems but is currently abstinent.
- The patient with no past or current history but who exhibits atypical features in terms of description of the pain or medication usage (as described above).
- The patient with any of the above who has additional psychological or psychiatric problems.

It is useful to have the addiction service working side by side with physicians or surgeons at all times. This is especially true if they know the patient already. Thus, if the patient is stable or unstable on current treatment for addiction, contact with the prescribing doctor should be made as soon as possible. This will give some indication of the degree of severity of addiction and associated problems. It should be noted that instability in the substitution regimen may be a direct result of the painful condition, and an attempt to (self) manage it with opiates, so it is not necessarily a negative prognostic feature.

If the patient is not being treated by the substance misuse service, and once it becomes apparent that there are suspicions that there may be a problem, their advice should be sought as soon as possible. There is a need to try to prevent reinstatement of a previous addiction problem resulting from the treatment for pain.

Treatment for the painful condition should be instituted as soon as possible to stabilize the pain if it is of an acute nature e.g. fracture, and treatment for addiction should be continued as recommended by the prescribing service. If the pain is of a more chronic nature, it may be possible to titrate the dose required against the dose of prescribed medication e.g. methadone, until there is pain relief. Alternatively it may be appropriate to use additional medication to gain a degree of control over the pain, at least in the initial stages.

Methadone works well as an analgesic for neuropathic pain. Buprenorphine (Transtec® in lower doses patches compared to Subutex®) is used as an effective analgesic. The WHO analgesic ladder should not be discarded for addicted individuals and both opioids and non-opioids can be used with clear justifications. It is important to consider the dosage, frequency and route of administration and method of delivery (e.g. patches rather than tablets). Prescribing must be undertaken with minimal risk of abuse/overdose.

With careful monitoring of the pain control and dosage of combined medications e.g. methadone and morphine, it should be possible to determine to what extent addiction and pain is being controlled. There are scales available to assess degree of withdrawal, and the need for extra medication to control opiate misuse. After some time, when the acute painful condition has stabilized on medication, it may be possible to transfer to the equivalent dose of one medication only e.g. methadone, and then reduce it over time.

Thus it is vital that the initial and ongoing assessments should also include decisions about psychological and pharmacological treatments for those components, in addition to that for pain, and for addiction (Curran & Drummond, 2005; Pain Society *et al.* 2004; Wanigaratne *et al.* 2005). Such decisions should be made within the context of the patient's psychosocial environment so psychological approaches should be discussed and considered at the same time as pharmacological. Of course, this has to be discussed with the patient and their family so that they do not have unrealistic expectations of medications and they can receive psychosocial support.

Plans for the regular review of the patient's condition should be made with the view to attempting to reduce analgesic medication and substitute medication. It may even result in eventual dosage reduction for any addiction problem at initial presentation.

8.10 Outcome studies in older people with substance problems

Several USA studies have found that treatment for substance misuse in older people works, so if patients in pain are identified as misusing drugs, outcome can be good. Satre *et al.* (2004) reported a five-year alcohol and drug treatment outcome study as a comparative study of older adults (aged 55–77) versus younger and middle aged people. They found that older adults were less likely to be drug dependent at baseline than younger (aged 18–39) and middle aged (aged 40–54) adults and had longer retention in treatment than younger adults. At five years, older adults were less likely than younger adults to have close family or friends who encouraged alcohol or drug use. Fifty-two percent of older adults had been totally abstinent from alcohol and drugs in the past 30 days, versus 40% of younger adults. Older women had higher 30-day abstinence rates than older men or younger women. This data provides valuable information on which to base service provision, e.g. persistence in treatment has long lasting benefits, the need for adequate social support, less likelihood of encouragement to use substances from family and friends. Satre *et al.* (2003) also demonstrated that older patients are more likely to have an abstinence goal and a lower rate of psychiatric symptoms than younger people (Oslin *et al.* 2002; Satre *et al.* 2003). Brennan *et al.* (2003) also found that older substance misusers were less likely to be experiencing drug problems and psychiatric problems, but more likely to report alcohol and medical problems, and had better outcomes than a matched sample of younger patients.

There are very few publications that have concentrated on the treatment of older people in isolation. Box 8.6 provides some additional references as examples, but most are comparisons.

8.11 Conclusions

There is a vastly more enhanced evidence base on which to draw for better epidemiological data and the effectiveness of treatment interventions for alcohol, nicotine and opiates. Even the National Service Framework for Older People (Department of Health, 2001) did not acknowledge that addiction was of relevance for older people. There is no dedicated specialist substance misuse service in the UK for provision for older people. Older people in pain remain an invisible, hidden, stigmatized and neglected group, which is being 'misused' in the sense that they are not being exposed to, or evaluated on, the rapidly developing treatment portfolio for substance misusers.

Box 8.6 Further reading relating to the treatment of older people

Appel DW and Aldrich TK (2003). Smoking cessation in the elderly. *Clinics in Geriatric Medicine*, **19**, 77–100.

Blow. FC. (2000). Treatment of older women with alcohol problems: Meeting the challenge for a special population. *Alcoholism: Clinical and Experimental Research*, **24**, 1257–66.

Brennan PL, Kagay CR, Geppert JJ, *et al.* (2000). Elderly medicare in patients with substance use disorders: Characteristics and predictors of hospital readmissions over a four–year interval. *Journal of Studies on Alcohol*, **61**, 891–5.

Dale L, Olsen D, Patten C, *et al.* (1997). Predictors of smoking cessation among elderly smokers treated for nicotine dependence. *Tobacco Control*, **6**, 181–7.

Dupree LW, Broskowski H and Schonfeld L (1984). The Gerontology Alcohol Project: A behavioural treatment program for elderly alcohol abusers. *The Gerontologist*, **24**, 510–16.

Firoz S and Carlson G (2004). Characteristics and treatment outcome of older methadone-maintenance patients. *American Journal of Geriatric Psychiatry*, **12**, 539–41.

Fleming M (2002). Identification and treatment of alcohol use disorders in older adults. In *Treating Alcohol and Drug Abuse in the Elderly* (eds Gurnack AM, Atkinson R and Osgood N J), pp.85–108. Springer Publishing Company, New York.

Kaempf G, O'Donnell C, and Oslin DW (1999). The BRENDA model: A psychosocial addiction model to identify and treat substance misuse in elders. *Geriatric Nursing*, **20**, 302–4.

Lemke S, and Moos RH, (2003) Outcomes at 1 and 5 years for older patients with alcohol use disorders. *Journal of Substance Abuse Treatment*, **24**, 43–50.

Miller NS, Belkin BM, and Gold MS (1991). Alcohol and drug dependence among the elderly: Epidemiology, diagnosis and treatment. *Comprehensive Psychiatry*, **32**, 153–65.

Oslin D, Liberto JG, O'Brien J, *et al.* (1997). Naltrexone as an adjunctive treatment for older patients with alcohol dependence. *American Journal of Geriatric Psychiatry*, **5**, 324–32.

Schonfeld L, (2005). The Florida BRITE project. In *Substance Abuse Amongst Seniors: New Research Developments and Innovations* (Workshop presented at the Joint Conference of the American Society on Aging and the National Council on Aging) (Chair F. Blow). Philadelphia, PA.

Box 8.7 Learning points for management of older substance users (Adapted from Raw *et al.* 1998)

1) Ask
- Ask all patients about their history and record the findings
- Style is a powerful determinant
- Be aware of and sensitive to ambivalence
- Be non-judgemental
- Use a non-confrontational style

2) Assess
- Is there a degree of dependence or not?
- Should be a thorough, ongoing assessment and include a comprehensive history
- Neurocognitive impairment
- Semi-structured interviews increase identification
- There are many tools for screening, assessment and monitoring outcome
- Assess severity of substance use, misuse, or dependence
- Educate the patient about withdrawal
- Assess motivation and stage of change
- Goals—advice on cessation or (harm) reduction
- Treatment choice and appropriateness—pharmacological interventions
- Specialised services—admission

3) Advise—brief intervention
- 5–10 minutes duration
- Motivational interviewing techniques
- Information and education—personal benefits/risks
- Information about safe levels, e.g. drinking
- Advise on ways to stop smoking and reduce drinking or use of medications or illicit drugs
- Harm reduction approach
- Provision of self-help materials
- Ventilation of anxieties and other problems
- Personalized feedback about results of screening/blood tests

4) Assist
- Offer support and encouragement
- Instil positive expectations of success
- If there have been previous attempts to quit or cut down, the patient may be low in confidence

Box 8.7 (*Contd.*)

- Set a 'quit date' and decide on a goal—abstinence or reduction
- Get rid of substances
- Offer a 'menu' of alternative coping strategies
- Identify cues: distract, escape, avoid, delay

5) Admission

- Severe physical illness
- Comorbid severe mental illness, e.g. depression
- Abuse multiple substances, including over the counter medications and are poorly compliant with prescribed medications
- Frequent relapses
- Patients with unstable social circumstances, e.g. living alone.

Box 8.8 Learning points: Unique treatment needs of older adults (US Dept of Health & Human Services, 1998)

- Emphasis on age-specific rather than mixed-age treatment
- Use of supportive, nonconfrontational approaches that build self-esteem
- Focus on cognitive-behavioural approaches to address negative emotional states such as depression, loneliness and feelings of loss
- Development of skills for improving social support
- Recruitment of counsellors trained and motivated to work with older adults
- Capacity to provide referrals to medical, mental health and aging services
- Appropriate pace and content for older adults

Box 8.9 Learning points: guidance for carers (adapted from US Dept of Health & Human Services, 2005)

- Cultivate the patient's self-esteem and confidence
- Take into account the older person's perceptual needs, for example with regards to terminology
- Take any cognitive impairment into account
- Be aware of literacy and language needs
- Be aware of sensory needs and sensory decline in the older person

References

Adams LL, Gatchel RJ, Robinson RC, *et al.* (2004). Development of a self-report screening instrument for assessing potential opioid medication misuse in chronic pain patients. *Journal of Pain and Symptom Management*, **27**, 440–59.

American Psychiatric Association (1994). *Diagnostic and statistical manual of mental disorders IV*. Washington DC: American Psychiatric Association.

Baptista A, Bianchi L, Groote JD, *et al.* (1981). Alcoholic liver disease: Morphological manifestations—Review by an international group. *Lancet*, **1**, 707–11.

Beresford TB (2000). Alcoholism. In *Oxford Textbook of Geriatric Medicine* (eds J. G. Williams TF, Williams BL, Beatie, *et al.*), Oxford University Press, Oxford, pp 1008–21.

Blow FC, Brower KJ, Schulenberg JE, *et al.* (1992). The Michigan Alcoholism Screening Test – Geriatric Version (MAST-G): A new elderly-specific screening instrument. *Alcoholism: Clinical and Experimental Research*, **16**, 372.

Bouckoms AJ, Masand P, Murray GB, *et al.* (1992). Chronic non-malignant pain treated with long-term oral narcotic analgesics. *Annals of Clinical Psychiatry*, **4**, 85–92.

Brennan PL, Nichol AC, and Moos RH (2003). Older and younger patients with substance use disorders: Outpatient mental health service use and functioning over a 12-month interval. *Psychology of Addictive Behaviors*, **17**, 42–8.

Brennan PL, Schutte KK, and Moos RH (2005). Pain and use of alcohol to manage pain: Prevalence and 3-year outcomes among older problem and non-problem drinkers. *Addiction*, **100**, 777–86.

Chabal C, Erjavec MK, Jacobson L, *et al.* (1997). Prescription opiate abuse in chronic pain patients: Clinical criteria, incidence and predictors. *Clinical Journal of Pain*, **13**, 150–5.

Chrischilles EA, Lemke JH, Wallace RB, *et al.* (1990). Prevalence and characteristics of multiple analgesic drug use in an elderly study group. *Journal of the American Geriatrics Society*, **38**, 979–84.

Compton P, Darakjian J, and Miotto K (1998). Screening for addiction in patients with chronic pain and "problematic" substance use: Evaluation of a pilot assessment tool. *Journal of Pain and Symptom Management*, **16**, 355–63.

Cook CC, Hallwood PM, and Thomson AD (1998). B vitamin deficiency and neuropsychiatric syndromes in alcohol misuse. *Alcohol and Alcoholism*, **33**, 317–36.

Coulthard M, Farrell M, Singleton N, *et al.* (2002). *Tobacco, alcohol and drug use and mental health*. The Stationery Office, London.

Cowan DT, Wilson-Barnett J, Griffiths P, *et al.* (2005). A randomised, double-blind, placebo-controlled, cross-over pilot study to assess the effects of long-term opioid drug consumption and subsequent abstinence in chronic noncancer pain patients receiving controlled-release morphine. *Pain Medicine*, **6**, 113–21.

Crome IB (1999). Substance misuse and psychiatric comorbidity: Towards improved service provision. *Drugs: Education, Prevention and Policy*, **6**, 154–71.

Crome I, and Bloor R, (in press a) Alcohol problems. In *Essentials in Psychiatry* (eds R. Murray, K. S. Kendler, P. McGuffin *et al.*). Cambridge: Cambridge University Press.

Crome I, and Bloor R (2006) Older substance misusers *still* deserve better diagnosis—An update (Part 2). *Reviews in Clinical Gerontology*, **15**, 255–62.

Crome IB and Ghodse A H (in press). Drug misuse in medical patients. In *Handbook of Liaison Psychiatry* Lloyd G, and Guthrie E, (eds). Cambridge University Press, Cambridge.

Cuijpers P, Riper H, and Lemmers L (2004). The effects on mortality of brief interventions for problem drinking: A meta-analysis. *Addiction*, **99**, 839–45.

Curran V, and Drummond C (2005). *Psychological treatments of substance misuse and dependence*. Foresight, London.

Department of Health (2001). *National service framework for older people*. Department of Health, London.

Ewing JA (1984). Detecting alcoholism: The CAGE questionnaire. *Journal of the American Medical Association*, **252**, 1905–07.

Fleming MF, Manwell LB, Barry KL, *et al.* (1999). Brief physician advice for alcohol problems in older adults: A randomised community-based trial. *Journal of Family Practice*, **48**, 378–84.

Friedman R, Li V, and Mehrotra D (2003). Treating pain patients at risk: Evaluation of a screening tool in opioid–treated pain patients with and without addiction. *Pain Medicine*, **4**, 182–5.

Gordon AJ, Conigliaro J, Maisto SA, *et al.* (2003). Comparison of consumption effects of brief interventions for hazardous drinking elderly. *Substance Use and Misuse*, **38**, 1017–35.

Gossop M, Marsden J, Stewart D, *et al.* (2003). The National Treatment Outcome Research Study (NTORS): 4-5 year follow-up results. *Addiction*, **98**, 291–303.

Gottlieb S (2004). Inappropriate drug prescribing in elderly people is common. *British Medical Journal*, **329**, 367.

Graham K, Carver V, and Brett PJ (1995). Alcohol and drug use by older women: Results of a national survey. *Canadian Journal on Ageing*, **14**, 769–91.

Jaffe J (1992). Opiates: Clinical aspects. In *Substance Abuse: A Comprehensive Text* (eds Lowinson J, Ruiz P, Millman R, *et al.*), Williams & Wilkins, Baltimore, pp. 186–94.

Jamison RN, Anderson KO, Peeters-Asdourian C, *et al.* (1994). Survey of opioid use in chronic non-malignant pain patients. *Regional Anesthesia*, **19**, 225–30.

Kelly KD, Pickett W, Yiannakoulias N, *et al.* (2003). Medication use and falls in community dwelling older persons. *Age and Ageing*, **32**, 503–9.

Kouyanou K, Pither CE, and Wessely S (1997). Medication misuse, abuse and dependence in chronic pain patients. *Journal of Psychosomatic Research*, **43**, 497–504.

Lingford-Hughes AR, Welch S, and Nutt DJ (2004). Evidence-based guidelines for the pharmacological management of substance misuse, addiction and comorbidity: Recommendations from the British Association for Psychopharmacology. *Journal of Psychopharmacology*, **18**, 293–335.

Littlejohn C, Baldacchino A, and Bannister J (2004). Chronic non-cancer pain and opioid dependence. *Journal of the Royal Society of Medicine*, **97**, 62–5.

Lynskey MT, Day C, and Hall W (2003). Alcohol and other drug use disorders among older people. *Drug and Alcohol Review*, **22**, 125–33.

Mayfield D, McLeod G, and Hall P (1974). The CAGE questionnaire: Validation of a new alcoholism screening instrument. *American Journal of Psychiatry*, **131**, 1121–3.

McLellan AT, Hagan TA, Levine M, *et al.* (1999). Does clinical case management improve outpatient treatment? *Drug and Alcohol Dependence*, **55**, 91–103.

McGrath A, Crome P, and Crome IB (2005). Substance misuse in the older population. *Postgraduate Medicine*, **81**, 228–31.

Michna E, Ross EL, Hynes WL, *et al.* (2004). Predicting aberrant drug behaviour in patients treated for chronic pain: Importance of abuse history. *Journal of Pain and Symptom Management*, **28**, 250–8.

Moore AA, Morton SC, Beck JC, *et al.* (1999). A new paradigm for alcohol use in older persons. *Medical Care*, **37**, 165–79.

Mundt MP, French MT, Roebuck MC, *et al.* (2005). Brief physician advice for problem drinking among older adults: An economic analysis of costs and benefits. *Journal of Studies on Alcohol*, **66**, 389–94.

Nguyen K, Fink A, Beck JC, *et al.* (2001). Feasibility of using an alcohol-screening and health education system with older primary care patients. *Journal of the American Board of Family Practitioners*, **14**, 7–15.

Office for National Statistics (2001). *Living in Britain 2001 – Supplementary report: People aged 65 and over.* Office for National Statistics, London.

Oslin DW, Pettinati H, and Volpicelli JR (2002). Alcoholism treatment adherence: Older age predicts better adherence and drinking outcomes. *American Journal of Geriatric Psychiatry*, **10**, 740–7.

Ozdemir V, Fourie J, Busto U, *et al.* (1996). Pharmacokinetic changes in the elderly: Do they contribute to drug abuse and dependence? *Clinical Pharmacokinetics*, **31**, 372–85.

Pain Society, Royal College of Anesthetists, Royal College of General Practitioners, *et al.* (2004). *Recommendations for the appropriate use of opioids for persistent non-cancer pain.* The Pain Society, London.

Portenoy RK, and Payne R (1997). Acute and chronic pain. In *Substance Abuse: A Comprehensive Textbook* (eds Lowinson J, Ruiz P, Millman R, *et al.*), Williams & Wilkins, Baltimore, pp. 563–90.

Poschl G, and Seitz HK (2004). Alcohol and cancer. *Alcohol and Alcoholism*, **39**, 155–65.

Raw M, McNeill A, West R (1998). Smoking cessation guidelines for health professionals. A guide to effective smoking cessation interventions for the health care system. Thorax, **53** (Suppl 5, Pt 1), S1–19.

Satre DD, Mertens JR, Arean PA, *et al.* (2004). Five year alcohol and drug treatment outcomes of older adults versus middle aged and younger adults in a managed care program. *Addiction*, **99**, 1286–97.

Satre DD, Mertens JR, Arean PA, *et al.* (2003). Contrasting outcomes of older versus middle-aged and younger adult chemical dependency patients in a managed care program. *Journal of Studies on Alcohol*, **64**, 520–30.

Savage SR (1996). Long-term opioid therapy: Assessment of consequences and risks. *Journal of Pain and Symptom Management*, **11**, 274–86.

Schieffer BM, Pham Q, Labus J, *et al.* (2005). Pain medication beliefs and medication misuse in chronic pain. *Journal of Pain*, **6**, 620–9.

Sesso HD (2001). Alcohol and cardiovascular health: Recent findings. *American Journal of Cardiovascular Drugs*, **1**, 167–72.

Stack K, Cortina J, Samples C, *et al.* (2000). Race, age and back pain as factors in completion of residential substance abuse treatment by veterans. *Psychiatric Services*, **51**, 1157–61.

Stein MD (1997). Medical disorders in addicted patients. In *The Principles and Practice of Addictions in Psychiatry* Miller N (ed). WB. Saunders, Baltimore, pp.144–54.

Theodoulou M, Harriss L, Hawton K, *et al.* (2005). Pain and deliberate self harm: An important association. *Journal of Psychosomatic Research*, **58**, 317–20.

UKATT Research Team (2005). Effectiveness of treatment for alcohol problems: Findings of the randomised UK Alcohol Treatment Trial (UKATT). *British Medical Journal*, **331**, 527–8.

US Dept of Health & Human Services (2005). *Substance abuse relapse prevention for older adults.* Rockville: US Dept of Health & Human Services.

US Dept of Health & Human Services (1998). *Substance abuse among older adults* (Treatment Improvement Protocol (TIP) Series No. 26). Rockville: US Dept of Health & Human Services.

Wanigaratne S, Davis P, Pryce K, *et al.* (2005). *The effectiveness of psychological therapies on drug misusing clients* (Research briefing: 11). National Treatment Agency, London.

Whelan, G. (2003) Alcohol: A much neglected risk factor in elderly mental disorders. *Current Opinion in Psychiatry*, **16**, 609–14.

World Health Organization (1992). *ICD 10 classification of mental and behavioural disorders.* World Health Organization, Geneva.

Chapter 9

Cognitive behavioural therapy

Chris J. Main, Sandra J. Waters, and Francis J. Keefe

Key points

- Adopt a biopsychosocial perspective in which each component needs to be evaluated before developing a treatment plan.
- Centre recommendations on meaningful and age-appropriate goals, identified and agreed with the patient.
- Assess the possible influence of cognitive, auditory, visual, and physical impairments.
- Consider not only the content but also the *method* of information transmission.
- Be prepared to allow extra time/sessions to ensure comprehension, retention of information, and skills acquisition.
- Supplement discussion with the provision of reminders and encouragement in whatever form seems most appropriate for the patient.
- Continually emphasize the patient's ownership of the change process as a way of increasing the likelihood of maintaining and further developing treatment gains after the conclusion of treatment.
- If possible involve a family member or care-giver in the treatment plan.

9.1 Introduction and clarification of terms

9.1.1 The conceptual framework

Cognitive-behavioural therapy (CBT) in the treatment and management of pain is aligned with a biopsychosocial conceptualization of pain (Waddell 1987; White, 2005) in which pain is addressed from its biological, psychological, and social aspects, and the interactions among these facets is explicitly recognized (Turk *et al.* 1983). As an approach to therapy it has its origins within the mental health domain, where it is the treatment approach of choice for many mental health conditions.

9.1.2 Models of disease and illness

Within the area of pain management, the cognitive-behavioural approach (CBA) has allowed a broadening in view from the pathology or disease model which underpins much of medicine. Persistent pain and its spectrum of pain-associated limitations can not only significantly diminish quality of life but also lead to significant levels of distress requiring psychological or psychiatric treatment in its own right. The advent of the CBA however has allowed a much wider range of possibilities for intervention, derived from a systematic analysis of specific beliefs, emotional responses, and pain behaviour, and sits well with an approach to treatment which maximizes the patient's own engagement in, and responsibility for, the management of their own pain and its effects.

9.1.3 Essential features of the cognitive-behavioural approach (CBA)

Key assumptions underpinning CBA are shown in Box 9.1. In practical terms, CBA can be divided into two phases: assessment and treatment.

9.1.3.1 Assessment

The assessment phase of CBA is guided by a biopsychosocial model that maintains that pain is influenced by, and in turn influences, biological, psychological, and social factors. Initial assessment includes a review of medical records, semi-structured interviews, psychological testing, and behavioural observations. Structured daily pain diaries are also used as an initial and ongoing assessment method. These diaries typically require patients to make daily entries regarding relevant behaviours (e.g. uptime—time spent up and out of the reclining position), thoughts (e.g. negative thoughts about self, others, or the future), feelings (e.g. depression, anxiety), and pain (e.g. pain level on a scale of 0 = no pain to 10 = pain as bad as it can be). Pain diaries are useful initially in helping patients detect unhelpful thoughts and behaviours that may be contributing to psychological distress and exacerbating their pain experience. They also provide a very useful means of monitoring the effects of CBT.

9.1.3.2 Treatment

In the treatment phase of CBA patients are provided with a rationale for training in pain-coping skills such as the gate control theory

(Melzack & Wall, 1965). This theory highlights the influence that cognition, affect, and behaviour can have on pain. It also emphasizes the important role that patients can play in managing their own pain by learning and mastering cognitive and behavioural pain coping skills. Many older adults adhere to a biomedical model that views pain as a sensory signal solely influenced by underlying tissue damage. The gate control rationale is important because it helps older adults realize that pain is influenced not only by biological factors such as tissue damage or injury, but also by psychological factors such as a sense of mastery over pain and social factors such as strong family support. Older adults often respond quite positively to this rationale noting that it validates many of their own experiences with pain.

A major focus of the treatment phase of CBA is teaching specific strategies for controlling thoughts and behaviours that may be contributing to pain problems (Waters *et al.* 2002). Typically, patients are trained in the use of a 'menu' of multiple coping skills that includes relevant behavioural skills (e.g. activity pacing, relaxation training) and cognitive skills (e.g., imagery, cognitive restructuring). The notion of a 'menu' is important in that it suggests that multiple strategies are available, that the patient has choice over which strategies to use, and that the strategies can be used in different combinations. Training in pain coping skills typically is carried out in a series of six to ten individual or group sessions helping weekly. The format for these sessions involves setting an agenda, review of home practice, instruction in a specific skill, rehearsal of that skill, and identifying goals for home practice. An important goal of training is to help patients identify which coping skills work best for them, both in general and in response to specific situations.

Box 9.1 Key assumptions of the cognitive-behavioural approach

- Individuals are active processors of information and not passive reactors.
- Thoughts can influence and be influenced by mood, have social consequences, and can serve as an impetus for behaviour.
- Behaviour is reciprocally determined by both individual and environmental factors.
- Individuals can learn more adaptive ways of thinking feeling and behaving.
- Individuals should be active collaborative agents in changing their maladaptive thoughts feelings and behaviours.

Turk and Okifuji (2003), Table 36.1, p534.

9.1.4 **Range of applications**

CBT has been shown to be effective in a wide range of health conditions (both 'physical' and 'mental') and is of particular value in the management of pain, whether disease-related or 'benign' musculoskeletal conditions. The approach is being used increasingly for the management of pain in older adults (Keefe *et al.* 2002).

9.1.5 **Efficacy**

Although the CBA is the treatment of choice for chronic pain (Morley *et al.*1999) there have been few studies as yet of its efficacy with older adults. Given the sense of helplessness which frequently characterizes chronic pain, there is no reason *a priori* to suppose that an approach with its major focus on self-help should not be at least as effective, if not more effective, with older people.

9.2 Important considerations in using CBA with older adults

Waters *et al.* (2005) have identified a number of biological, psychological, and social challenges that are particularly important to consider when using CBA with older adults.

Among the most important biological factors are medical comorbidities (Waters, *et al.* 2005). Older adults who present with persistent pain often have multiple medical conditions, some of which contribute directly to their pain (e.g. osteoarthritis, musculoskeletal problems, cancer) and others which may contribute to their overall disability (e.g. heart disease). Thus, in older adults an identified pain problem often occurs in the context of multiple medical conditions. These comorbid conditions cause symptoms such as fatigue and insomnia that can exacerbate pain. Treatments for these conditions (e.g. cancer) also cause side effects (loss of appetite with weight loss) that may significantly interfere with behavioural and medical pain management efforts. As Waters *et al.* (2005) note, CBA is quite flexible and older adults often can be taught to apply learned pain coping skills to pain and other symptoms of their comorbid medical conditions.

Sensory changes such as hearing loss and visual impairments are common in older adults (Waters *et al.* 2005). Standard approaches to training in pain coping skills typically can be tailored on an individual basis to deal with these changes. For example, large type materials might be used with those having vision problems.

Cognitive declines occur in many older adults and can interfere with training in pain coping skills (Waters *et al.* 2005). These declines may be related to normal aging or to dementias such as Alzheimer's disease. Although there is some evidence for the value of CBT at early stages of dementia, the loss of faculty associated with advanced dementia represent a major impediment to CBT, although it has been shown to be of benefit in reduction of anxiety in caregivers.

Depression, anxiety, and fear all increase in prevalence with age and late-life depression is believed to be a primary cause of emotional distress and reduced quality of life (Blazer 2003; Jorsh, Chapter 10, this volume). In older adults with persistent pain, depression appears to exacerbate the impact of pain on physical functioning. This may present as frank helplessness, associated with lessening in self-confidence (lessening in self-efficacy beliefs). CBT may be helpful for managing both the pain and the depression. Among older people, pain-related anxiety is associated with depression. This may be fairly generalized (widespread) or may have a much narrower focus such as concerns about their pain getting out of control and their pain-associated limitations becoming unmanageable.

The belief that ageing is synonymous with physical and mental decline is still prevalent in society (Angus & Reeve, 2006; Lupien & Wan, 2004). The negative stereotypes formed by this belief influence the self-image and behaviours of older adults in many ways. For example, when negative age-related stereotypes are activated, older adults experience increases in cardiovascular arousal (Levy *et al.* 2000) and poorer memory performance (Hess *et al.* 2003). In addition, older adults often internalize negative age-related stereotypes (Levy, 2003) which may change self-perceptions, e.g. lower self-efficacy beliefs. Fortunately, self-efficacy can be raised using a cognitive-behaviour approach for teaching older adults strategies for coping with specific problems (e.g., coping with chronic pain; Lefebvre *et al.* 1999). It can be helpful to reframe emotionally loaded thoughts as cognitive distortions and adopt a CBT approach. Helping the patient to develop alternative cognitions, focusing on the 'next step' rather than the eventual outcome, and developing an implementation plan with small steps guaranteeing successes are useful psychological techniques.

For older adults, the social context of pain is particularly important (Waters *et al.* 2005). An important strategy in optimizing the success of a CBA may be to establish a degree of social support from family or caregivers. With increasing years, however, many older people find themselves living on their own which is a risk factor for depression (Prince *et al.* (2000). The combination places the older person at significant increased risk of psychiatric illness. In this situation the role of carers can be extremely important. Older adults are also affected by health-related stereotypes held by others. These stereotypes reflect characteristics that devalue the individual (e.g., declines in functional ability and increased dependence on others) and are often viewed as debilitating (Bloom *et al.* 1991). Older adults are aware that, in medical environments, both age-related and health-related stereotypes may influence judgements made about their capabilities (Auman *et al.* 2005). Even if older adult patients are capable of participating in treatment programs using a cognitive-behavioural approach, medical personnel may not offer them such options. When treatment programmes based on a cognitive-behavioural approach are offered, older adult patients are reluctant to participate for fear of justifying the negative age- and health-related stereotypes (Auman *et al.* 2005). In order to provide older adults with opportunities for receiving adjuvant forms of treatment for pain and other medical conditions, it becomes the responsibility of clinicians and others to refrain from making global judgements about older adults' performance on cognitive and/or behavioural tasks. Clinicians should take care to recognize and refute, whenever possible, the negative stereotypes that might be worrying their patients.

It is also important to educate health professionals about the potential negative effects of stereotyping and to encourage them to adopt an empirical stance in which they withhold judgements on the success or failure of CBA for a given patient until a trial of treatment is instituted.

9.3 Clinical service delivery

9.3.1 CBT in secondary and tertiary settings

Pain is the most frequent symptom in patients attending hospital, and the management of the symptom of pain during and after surgical interventions is a cornerstone of anaesthetic practice and the basis from which pain modality treatments were originally developed (Bonica, 1990) developed in the early anaesthetist-run pain clinics is an integral part of hospital care. The development of CBT for the treatment of chronic pain offers a new range of opportunities for the management of pain in older people, and the use of cognitive-behavioural interventions is increasing, but there is as yet little systematic research on the elderly population.

A similar therapeutic approach may be embedded within larger and more comprehensive interdisciplinary pain management programmes (Main & Spanswick, 2000). The primary objectives of such programmes are shown in Box 9.2.

9.3.2 Focus of interventions

In many pain management programmes (PMPs), there is a major focus on pain management in the context of employment but the majority of older people are not employed, but there is more to life than work, and a significant proportion of people will live for two or three decades after they retire from paid employment. The recent WHO emphasis on maximizing participation as an important health outcome (ICF, 2001) and interfaces well with CBT in its focus not only on pain but on its effects. It is important therefore to determine the specific impact of pain on the patient's life and well-being. Some recommendations regarding assessment are presented in Box 9.3.

Box 9.2 Primary objectives of cognitive-behavioural treatment programmes

- To combat demoralization by assisting patients to change their view of their pain and suffering from overwhelming to manageable.
- To teach patients coping strategies and techniques to help them to adapt and respond to pain and the resultant problems.
- To assist patients to reconceptualize themselves as active, resourceful and competent.
- To learn the associations between thoughts, feelings, and their behaviour, and subsequently to identify and alter automatic, maladaptive patterns.
- To utilize these more adaptive responses.
- To bolster self-confidence and attribute successful outcomes to their own efforts.
- To help patients anticipate problems proactively and generate solutions, thereby facilitating maintenance and generalization.

Turk and Okifuji (2003), Table 36.3, p535.

Box 9.3 Recommendations regarding assessment

- Consider the person not just in terms of their pain, but in terms of their quality of life and social network.
- Consider possible cognitive, sensory, and physical factors which may compromise the person's understanding of what is said.
- Take a careful developmental history; of pain illness, and well-being.
- Include identification or recently valued activities.
- Focus on the biological, psychological, and social facets of their pain and functioning.
- Investigate the possibility of primary mental health problems, particularly depression and anxiety.
- Appraise their understanding of their pain and its implications for them.
- Obtain as much detail as possible about their social network, including family, and carers with a view to increase the chance of designing an effective intervention.

9.3.3 Multi- and interdisciplinary working

The nature and extent of treatment provision for pain management appears to be widely variable. If the patient has the benefit of access to multi- and interdisciplinary pain programmes, the blending of professional expertise may permit the design of an effective CBT intervention, but particular attention should be paid to ensuring a consistent and appropriately paced approach is offered to the patient. Even a fairly straightforward intervention may be viewed as a challenge and patients can become flustered and distressed if they have to cope with mixed or inconsistent messages. Careful and effective case management, by an identified member of the team assigned to the particular patient can go some way to guard against this potential problem.

9.3.4 CBT in community settings

9.3.4.1 *Access to treatment*

There can be also significant logistical and practical difficulties confronting the older patient in access seeking treatment. Access to and affording transport may be an important barrier to treatment. Travelling may place an additional burden on the already distressed chronic pain patient and so there are considerable advantages to community based services.

9.3.4.2 *Residential homes and day care facilities*

A proportion of patients live in residential homes and it can be assumed that a high proportion of such residents will have pain problems, particularly arthritis. Frequently chronic pain is viewed simply as an aspect of the ageing process and patients may suffer unnecessarily, particularly if they are cognitively impaired or behaviourally disinhibited. In such cases a self-directed CBT approach may be inappropriate, but involvement of a staff member as the key instigator of behavioural change may lead to improvement in overall pain management.

Similarly for patients attending day care centres there may be opportunities for involving staff in the design and delivery of CBT interventions, but the success of any such interventions will depend on a detailed and competent initial assessment as well as the requisite level of skill in the staff delivering the intervention.

9.3.4.3 *Domiciliary CBT*

Domiciliary CBT may be the preferred option for the patient. Unfortunately such services are not always available. However assessment of the patient in his/her own environment will give the professional a much clearer idea of the impact of chronic pain and opportunities for instigation of a CBT programmes. There may be an opportunity also to meet with carers and other members of the patient's social support network. Minimizing the inconvenience to the patient in this way, and obviating the dangers of interruption to a treatment programme as a consequence of difficulties in attending appointments are obvious additional advantages.

9.4 Issues of skills and training

9.4.1 Health-care professionals

CBT is a systematic therapeutic intervention and not just a matter of common sense. Specific training, including case-supervision, is required for accreditation. Different countries have different regulations in this matter.

CBT is recognized as a form of psychotherapy. In the UK, CBT as originally developed, appeared in the therapeutic armamentarium of health-care professionals such as clinical psychologists and psychiatrists. There are now accredited courses in CBT and an increasing number of other health-care professionals such as nurses and OTs are now obtaining such qualifications. It appears at present however that the emphasis principally is on CBT as applied to mental health problems such as anxiety or depression rather than to pain as such.

9.4.2 Generic workers

It is clear that there will never be enough specialists to deliver CBT to all patients with chronic pain, even were that desirable or appropriate. It may be, however, that something less than a full-blown CBT programme may be helpful. Giving the frequency of interactions between patients and staff there certainly is an opportunity of a more systematic approach to pain management. Better recognition of pain and its effects, particularly in those whose pain is perhaps masked by other more florid symptoms, might help to decrease suffering but a systematic approach should not be undertaken without establishment of appropriate competencies.

9.4.3 Carers

Involving family members or caregivers can be particularly beneficial. Caregivers involved in treatment are more likely to encourage or help older adults to attend sessions and encourage them in their homework. Keefe *et al.* (1996, 2001) demonstrated better outcomes for spouse-assisted coping skills training compared with training without spouse involvement or with the simple provision of educational information.

9.5 Conclusions

CBT is now well-recognized as an effective approach in pain management, whether delivered as the major or sole intervention, or whether as an adjunct to specific biomedical interventions. Research to date has primarily focused on non-elderly populations and as a consequence the potential of CBT as a self-directed approach perhaps has not as yet been fully realised in the management of pain in older people. Given the well-recognized psychological and social impact of pain in this population, this oversight must be addressed. It is important however to customize the content and manner of delivery of interventions to take account of potential dificulties in comprehension, information retention, and skills acquisition which may be particularly problematic in this group.

References

Angus J, Reeve P (2006). Ageism: A threat to "aging well" in the 21st century. *Journal of Applied Gerontology*, **25**, 137–52.

Auman C, Bosworth HB, and Hess TM (2005). Effect of health-related stereotypes on physiological responses of hypertensive middle-aged and older men. *Journal of Gerontology: Psychological sciences*, **60B**, 3–10.

Blazer DG (2003). Depression in later life: review and commentary. *J Geront Series A. Biol Sci and Med Sci*, **58**, M249–M265.

Bloom J, Grazier K, Hodge F, *et al.* (1991). Factors affecting the use of screening mammography among African American Women. *Cancer Epidemiology, Biomarkers, and Prevention*, **11**, 75–82.

Bonica JJ (1990). History of pain concepts and therapies. In J.J. Bonica (ed) *The Management of Pain* 2nd edn. Lea & Febiger, New York.

Hess TM, Auman C, Colcombe SJ, *et al.* (2003). The impact of stereotype threat on age differences in memory performance. *Journal of Gerontology: Psychological sciences*, **58B**, 3–11.

ICF (International Classification of Functioning, Disability and Health) (2001), World Health Organization, Geneva.

Keefe FJ, Caldwell DS, and Baucom D, (1996). Spouse-assisted coping skills training in the management of osteoarthritic knee pain. *Arthritis Care Research*, **9**, 279–91.

Keefe FJ, Caldwell DS, and Baucom D (2001). Spouse-assisted coping skills training in the management of osteoarthritic knee pain: longterm follow-up results. *Arthritis Care Research*, **12**, 101–11.

Lefebvre JC, Keefe FJ, Affleck G. *et al.* (1999). The relationship of arthritis self-efficacy to daily pain, daily mood, and daily pain coping in rheumatoid arthritis patients. *Pain*, **80**, 425–35.

Levy BR (2003). Mind matters: cognitive and physical effects of aging self-stereotypes. *The Journals of Gerontology Series B: Psychological Sciences and Social Sciences*, **58**, 203–11.

Levy BR, Hausdorff JM Hencke R, *et al.* (2000). Reducing cardiovascular stress with positive self-stereotypes of aging. *The Journals of Gerontology Series B: Psychological Sciences and Social Sciences*, **55**, 205–13.

Lupien SJ, and Wan N (2004). Successful ageing: from cell to self. *Phil Trans R Soc Lond* B, **359**, 1413–26.

Main CJ and Spanswick CC (2000). *Pain management: An Interdisciplinary Approach.* Churchill Livingstone, Edinburgh.

Melzack R and Wall PD (1965). Pain mechanisms: a new theory. *Science*, **150**, 971–79.

Morley SJ, Eccleston C, and Williams A (1999). Systematic Review And Meta-Analysis Of Randomised Controlled Trials Of Cognitive Behavioural Therapy And Behaviour Therapy For Chronic Pain In Adults. *Pain*, **80**, 1–13.

Prince MJ, Harwood RH, Blizard RA, *et al.* (2000). Social supports deficits, loneliness and life events as risk factors for depression in old age. *Psychol Med*, **27**, 323–32.

Turk DC, Meichenbaum DH, and Genest M (1983). *Pain And Behavioral Medicine: A Cognitive-Behavioral Perspective.* The Guilford Press, New York.

Turk DC and Okifuji A (2003). A Cognitive-Behavioral Approach To Pain Management. In Melzack R and Wall PD (eds) *Handbook Of Pain Management; A Clinical Companion To Wall And Melzack's Textbook Of Pain.* Churchill Livingstone, Edinburgh. pp.533–41.

Waddell G (1987). Volvo award in clinical sciences. A new clinical model for the treatment of low-back pain. *Spine*, **12**, 632–44.

Waters SJ, McKee DC, and Keefe FJ (2002). Cognitive behavioural approaches to the treatment of pain. *Trends in Evidence-based Neuropsychiatry*, **4**, 57–63.

Waters SJ, Woodward JT, and Keefe FJ (2005). Cognitive-behavioral therapy for pain in older adults. In Gibson SJ, Weiner DK (eds.). *Pain in Older Persons, Progress in Pain Research and Management*, **35**, 239–61. I.A.S.P. Press, Seattle.

White P (ed) (2005). *Biopsychosocial Medicine: an integrated approach to understanding illness.* Oxford University Press, Oxford.

Chapter 10

Depression and pain

Andy Moore and Mike Jorsh

Key points

- Pain is subjective and involves not just physical sensation but also affective, cognitive, and behavioural components.
- The aetiology of depression is multifactorial, and pain may be a highly significant contributing factor to a depressive episode.
- Depression more commonly follows pain than vice-versa, though pain experience can be modified by depression whatever the temporal sequence.
- Depression, like other forms of psychological distress, can be expressed as pain, through as yet unknown mechanisms.
- Management of comorbid pain and depression must be holistic, with attention given to both physical and emotional aspects of the patient.
- Whilst treatment of both chronic pain and depression needs to be tailored to take account of older age (e.g. drug doses), the underlying principles of treating both together are predominantly the same regardless of age.

10.1 Introduction

Individually, both depression and pain (usually chronic) in the elderly can present a considerable challenge to the clinician, but together that challenge can seem more than the sum of its parts. The intertwining of the two can at times be complex, requiring a detailed assessment of both, and their interplay in that particular patient, before a successful management strategy can be devised. Approaching such patients with a sound theoretical knowledge base should engender in the clinician a therapeutic optimism, rather than the foreboding that can so easily accompany such a potentially intimidating combination of problems.

10.1.1 **Components of pain**

Pain is a subjective and multidimensional experience, involving not just the noxious physical sensations, but also the associated affective, cognitive and behavioural components (Box 10.1). Historically, the physical sensory aspect has dominated both clinical and research attention, but recently, knowledge and clinical effort in the other dimensions have also increased. The importance of the emotional component was formally recognized in the definition of pain by the International Association for the Study of Pain (Merskey and Bogduk, 1994): 'an unpleasant sensory and *emotional experience* associated with actual or potential tissue damage, or described in terms of such damage' (italics added). More recently, advances in cognitive behavioural therapy techniques (both for pain and depression) have brought the remaining components into the picture. Increasing knowledge of peripheral pain pathways, and central processing (especially via functional neuroimaging) have confirmed the widely distributed nature of neural networks involved in pain, with significant representation from frontal (cognitive) and limbic (affective) areas amongst others, in both perceiving and modulating painful stimuli.

10.1.2 **Interaction of pain and depression**

Each of these four components (Box 10.1) can contribute to, or interact with, psychiatric illness in some way, depending on the individual circumstances. This could be as a predisposing factor (alone or with others), a direct causal precipitant, or a maintaining or exacerbating factor of pre-existing illness. The emotional aspect may seem the most prominent in psychiatric illnesses, but other dimensions are important too: depression can be thought of as a cognitive, as well as an affective disorder, and clearly also has a behavioural element. The picture becomes increasingly complex when it is recognized that the direction of influence between pain and emotions/mental illness can work both ways, with a range of possible mechanisms and temporal relationships.

Box 10.1 The four components of pain

- Physical/somatosensory
- Cognitive
- Affective
- Behavioural

This chapter will explore these issues with respect to depression, discuss the clinical management of comorbid pain and depression and finally look briefly at the theoretical ways that pain and depression can influence each other.

Figure 10.1 **Aetiological factors of depression**

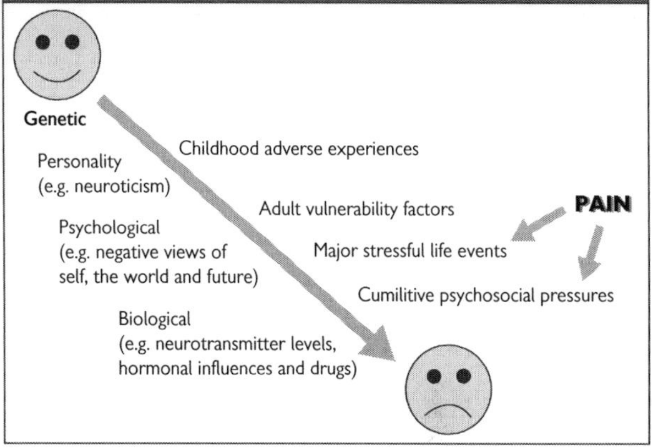

10.2 Causes of depression

Depression has a multifactorial aetiology. Each individual will have their own threshold for developing depression, with both genetic and environmental influences being important. These can occur, and exert themselves at various life stages, as illustrated above. Pain, possibly along with the originating illness, can be viewed as a major stressful life-event or a cumulative pressure, thus contributing to the process. The elderly have many years in which to gather vulnerability factors (as well as chronic painful conditions), and even though they may have occurred a long time previously they may still come into play given the right trigger factor.

10.3 Diagnosis of depression in the context of pain

10.3.1 Normal reactions to pain

Pain may be classified by timescale and is normally influenced by, and evokes a range of immediate emotions and longer lasting mood states, examples of which are given in Figure 10.2.

These may be adaptive in encouraging either actively defensive or more passive recovery-orientated behaviour as appropriate to the circumstances. These themselves will be mediated by cognitive appraisal of the circumstances and memory of past experience. The

Figure 10.2 Normal reactions to pain

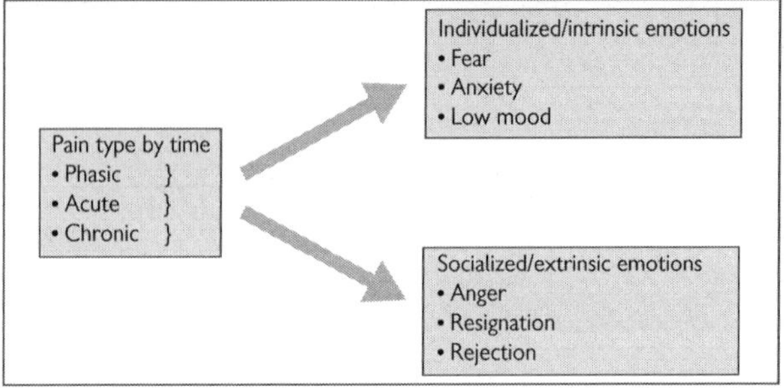

result of this complex mix is almost universally subjective distress for the individual, usually evident to others. The dilemma for the clinician is to distinguish between normal adaptive responses and pathology requiring intervention.

10.3.2 **Diagnosis of depression**

The diagnosis of depression requires a complete history and mental state examination. Screening tools such as the Hospital Anxiety and Depression Score, or Beck's Depression Inventory can assist, but do not replace this process. A clinical depressive episode is typically characterized by a persistent low mood lasting at least 2 weeks, which patients themselves can often qualitatively distinguish from transient 'unhappiness'; it tends to be more extreme and relentless, and accompanied by varying degrees of other symptoms and signs from the depressive spectrum, listed in Box 10.2.

10.3.3 **Problems with assessment**

Endicott (1984) noted that many of the recognized symptoms of depression were not applicable to the physically ill and therefore proposed modified diagnostic criteria for these individuals (see Box 10.3). The process of assessing whether an individual is suffering from depression or one of the 'milder' depressive spectrum disorders such as adjustment disorder or dysthymia can be complicated even further in the elderly if the patient has problems expressing themselves, for example because of dementia, or has other comorbid conditions (e.g. Parkinson's). In addition, reduced sleep and appetite may be a part of the normal aging process, but it is the recent change in these that should alert the clinician.

Box 10.2 Typical symptoms and mental state findings of a depressive episode

Symptoms

- Persistent low mood (often with diurnal variation: worse in mornings)
- Fatigue
- Anhedonia (inability to enjoy things)
- Poor concentration
- Irritability
- Guilt feelings
- Low self-esteem and confidence
- Disturbed sleep pattern (too little or too much)
- Lack of appetite
- Weight loss
- Loss of libido
- Thoughts of suicide and death

Mental state findings

- Looks unhappy and depressed
- Lacking usual degree of self-care
- Psychomotor agitation or retardation
- Speech may be reduced in amount and speed, and monotonous
- Cognitive distortions e.g. pessimistic thinking, overgeneralization
- Delusions and/or hallucinations in severe depression

Anxiety is a common accompanying symptom, but does not form part of the usual diagnostic criteria.

Box 10.3 Endicott criteria for depression in the medically ill

- *Fearful or depressed appearance
- *Social withdrawal or decreased talkativeness
- Psychomotor retardation or agitation
- Depressed mood, subjective or observed
- Marked diminished interest or pleasure in most activities, most of the day
- *Brooding, self-pity, or pessimism
- Feelings of worthlessness or excessive or inappropriate guilt
- Recurrent thoughts of death or suicide
- *Mood is non-reactive to environmental events

Five out of nine symptoms for at least two weeks

* These four symptoms replace:

(a) significant weight loss or gain (>5% of body weight); (b) insomnia or hypersomnia; (c) fatigue or loss of memory; (d) diminished ability to think or concentrate, or indecisiveness.

10.4 Treatment of depression

10.4.1 Holistic approach

Treatment options are considered in the light of the patient's individual circumstances. The condition must be treated holistically alongside the pain and associated factors; if either is overlooked therapeutic efforts may fail. Symptoms may interact in a systematized manner, which can be both advantageous (e.g. may be able to change one symptom by targeting another) and disadvantageous (a symptom may seem to improve, but actually 'reappear' in a different form). Other alternative or co-morbid diagnoses should also be considered, such as anxiety disorders, or substance misuse.

10.4.2 Treatment options

Treatment of any depressive episode is similar to that of a patient without pain, with a few specific concerns, especially in the elderly. Treatment tends to follow a 'stepped' approach depending on the severity of the depression, and excellent national guidelines from the National Institute of Clinical Excellence (NICE) now exist which cover all aspects of treatment (regardless of age.) These are summarized in Figure 10.3.

Figure 10.3 NICE 'stepped care' guidelines for the treatment of depression

STEP 1: Recognition in primary care and general hospital settings

STEP 2: Treatment of mild depression in primary care

STEP 3: Treatment of moderate to severe depression in primary care

STEP 4: Treatment of depression in mental health specialists

STEP 5: Inpatient treatment for depression

	Who is responsible for care?	What is the focus?	What do they do?
STEP 5:	Inpatient care, crisis teams	Risk to life, severe self-neglect	Medication, combined treatments, ECT
STEP 4:	Mental health specialists, inducing crisis teams	Treatment-resistant, recurrent, atypical and psychotic depression, and those at significant risk	Medication, complex psychological interventions, combined treatments
STEP 3:	Primary care team, primary care mental health worker	Moderate or severe depression	Medication, psychological interventions, social support
STEP 2:	Primary care team, primary care mental health worker	Mild depression	Watchful waiting, guided self-help, computerized CBT, exercise, brief psychological interventions
STEP 1:	GP, practice nurse	Recognition	Assessment

Figure 10.3 is reproduced from NICE Guideline CG23: '*Depression*', (2004), http://guidance.nice.org.uk/page.aspx?0=236667, with permission.

Of the psychotherapies, cognitive behavioural therapy (CBT) can be particularly useful, as it can be adapted to tackle both depression and pain. Selective serotonin reuptake inhibitors (SSRIs) tend to be the first antidepressant medication of choice due to their relative lack of side effects compared to the older 'tricyclic' antidepressants, especially in older people who tend to be more prone to adverse effects. However, this must be balanced against the useful pain moderating effects (especially neuralgic pain) of some tricyclic antidepressants, notably amitryptilline. The analgesic effect of amitryptilline is achieved at much smaller doses than that required for depression (e.g.10–25mg, as opposed to 75–150mg), but can still cause troublesome side effects such as sedation. This can be particularly important in the elderly as it can increase risk of falls, hip fractures etc. Elderly patients are also more likely to have other medical conditions which necessitate tricyclics being used with caution, if at all, e.g cardiac disease, glaucoma, and urinary retention. A newer class of antidepressants is the serotonin and noradrenaline reuptake inhibitors, (SNRIs), one of which, duloxetine, seems in some cases to have similar analgesic qualities to amitryptilline, but with a side effect profile closer to the SSRIs, making it theoretically promising in the elderly depressed patient with pain (though experience with this drug is as yet limited).

10.4.3 **Other considerations**

Polypharmacy is common in the elderly, and it is important to consider co-administered drugs as they may interact with antidepressants, or have their own psychotropic side effects, e.g. benzodiazepines may induce depression. Other considerations may include family dynamics and social factors such as housing, and risk management issues such as self-neglect and suicide. In terminal illness, desire to hasten death has been shown to be more closely associated with depression than accompanying pain (Mystakidou *et al.* 2005; O'Mahony *et al.* 2005).

10.5 **The relationship between pain and depression**

10.5.1 **Epidemiology**

Both pain and depression are common conditions, and as such they can be expected to appear comorbidly in many people, a finding confirmed by research in elderly as well as younger patients (Fishbain *et al.* 1997). Studies looking at various populations of (mostly chronic) pain patients have found increased rates of mental illness compared with the general population, including double the lifetime rates for depression, and up to nine times the risk after age of pain onset. Interestingly, 'pre-pain-onset' depression rates have been found to be no different, whilst alcohol misuse rates can be raised (Atkinson *et al.* 1996). Previous history of depression does not seem as important as the pain itself, though it may lead to earlier onset of depression (Gallagher and Verma, 2004). Likewise, people with mental health problems have been noted to experience significant degrees of comorbid pain, depending on the population studied (Chaturvedi, 1987). Inconsistencies in research diagnostic criteria, along with heterogeneous study populations have led to wide variations in proportions quoted each way. It is worth noting that despite these findings, the majority of people with pain do not go on to develop depression. The positive association of pain with depression has been found to hold true in many different pain conditions, in several cultures, across the age range and in both sexes, though with some subtle variations in each of these (Fishbain *et al.* 1997; Gagliese and Melzack, 2003; Romano and Turner, 1985). This association may be particularly strong and direct in old age (Turk *et al.* 1995), and possibly more so in elderly men than women (Geerlings *et al.* 2002), implying a need for greater vigilance as increases in pain levels are more likely to lead to worsening depression, and vice-versa.

10.5.2 **Temporal relationship**

Research to date has shown that the commonest temporal relationship is for depression to follow pain, rather than vice versa, supporting a stronger causal relationship in that direction, with both presenting simultaneously in up to 50% in some studies (Atkinson *et al.* 1991; Gamsa, 1990). However, depression can still present first, or further influence pain in a form of 'positive feedback' loop. Add in the simultaneous possibility of exacerbating and confounding factors (e.g. disability) and a complex interactive picture emerges, summarized schematically in Figure 10.4.

The influence of past events and life stressors have already been mentioned in terms of causing depression, but they can directly affect pain perception too. Anticipatory anxiety can increase postoperative pain, whilst early experience and contextual factors will influence cognitive appraisal of pain, and the subsequent meaning and evaluation attached to it. Negative appraisals, especially those related to loss, may lead to depression. The initial acute phase of pain may be successfully negotiated with normal mental health, but ongoing chronicity, perhaps with accumulating social losses (e.g. job, mobility), whether as direct consequences of pain or via other related factors such as disability, may take their toll and lead to depression later. Studies have shown the importance of chronicity of pain in this respect, with one year being significant in one study population (Brown, 1990).

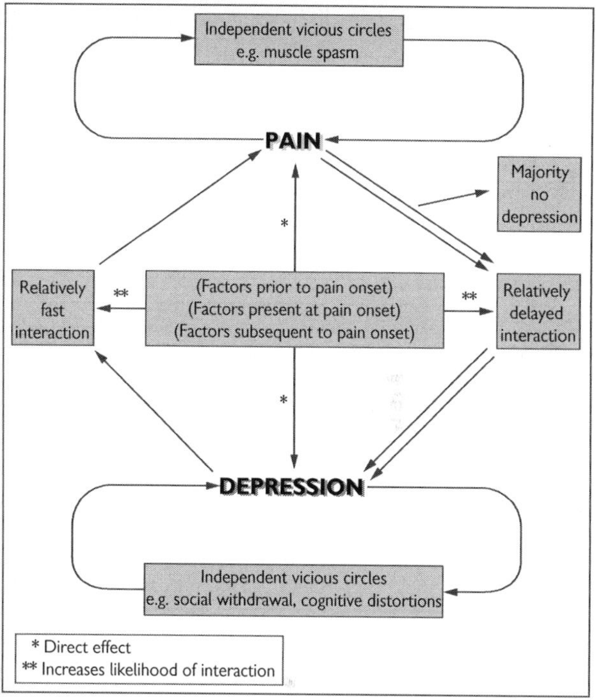

Figure 10.4 Schematic diagram representing the possible interactions of pain and depression, with confounding and exacerbating influences. The double arrows represent the finding that this is the commoner temporal relationship.

10.5.3 **Effect of depression on pain**

Studies have usually, though not invariably, demonstrated reduced experimental pain thresholds in depressed patients, and increased levels of pain reported with increasingly depressed populations. Five possible mechanisms of influence have been identified (Merskey, 1999), summarized in Box 10.4.

The first is via anxiety, which although not a specific symptom of depression is a common comorbid symptom, and usually increases subjective pain. In clinical practice reducing anxiety often reduces pain, possibly via the influence of higher brain function on the peripheral pain 'gateway' via descending fibres.

A second way of influence, again possibly more related to comorbid anxiety is via muscular 'tension pain' mechanisms, whereby increased muscle tone, especially in unexercised muscle, may directly give rise to pain.

Box 10.4 Possible mechanisms by which depression may influence pain

- Via comorbid anxiety
- Via increased muscular tension
- 'Hysterical' or 'Psychosomatic' mechanisms
- Hypochondriacal magnification
- Somatic hallucinations of pain (rare)

A third, and important way is via 'hysterical' or 'psychosomatic' mechanisms, in which it is proposed that psychological distress is converted to and expressed as physical symptoms such as pain. In clinical practice this requires more than merely an absence of identifiable physical causes, but also the positive presence of plausible psychological reasons, both proportional to the distress and temporally associated with it. Given the subjective nature of pain, it can be argued that the presence or absence of an identifiable organic cause is immaterial, and both research and clinical practice demonstrate the difficulty of confidently ruling out all possibility of organic causes.

Fourthly, hypochondriacal symptoms may be present in depression, and will tend to magnify any physical pain already present. Lastly, severe psychotic depression can very rarely present with somatic hallucinations of pain.

10.6 Conclusions

Pain and depression in all age groups presents a significant clinical challenge in its assessment and management, requiring a broad holistic approach. This is perhaps especially so with the older patient, who has a lifetime of influential experiences to consider, along with an increased likelihood of complicating physical comorbidity and psychosocial needs. The potential complexity of this task should not induce therapeutic pessimism, but rather vigorous, energetic attempts to identify the many potential ways in which these patients can be helped.

References

Atkinson JH, Slater MA, Patterson TL, *et al.* (1991). Prevalence, onset and risk of psychiatric disorders in men with chronic low back pain: a controlled study. *Pain*, **45**, 111–21.

Brown GK (1990). A causal analysis of chronic pain and depression. *Journal of Abnormal Psychology*, **99**, (2), 127–37.

Chaturvedi SK (1987). Prevalence of chronic pain in psychiatric patients. *Pain*, **29**, 231–7.

Endicott J. (1984). Measurement of depression in outpatients with cancer. *Cancer*, **53**, 2243–48.

Fishbain DA, Cutler RB, Rosomoff HL, *et al.* (1997). Chronic pain-associated depression: antecedent or consequence of chronic pain? A review. *Clinical Journal of Pain*, **13**, 116–37.

Gagliese L and Melzack R (2003). Age-related differences in the qualities but not the intensity of chronic pain. *Pain*, **104**, 597–608.

Gallagher KM and Verma S (2004). Mood and anxiety disorders in chronic pain. In Dworkin RH, Breilbart WS (eds). *Psychosocial aspects of pain: a handbook for healthcare providers.* IASP Press, Seattle, pp.139–79.

Gamsa A (1990). Is emotional disturbance a precipitator or a consequence of chronic pain? *Pain*, **42**, 183–95.

Geerlings SW, Twisk J, Beekman ATF, *et al.* (2002). Longitudinal relationship between pain and depression in older adults: sex, age and physical disability. *Social Psychiatry and Psychiatric Epidemiology*, **37**, 23–30.

Merskey H (1999). Pain and psychological medicine. In Wall PD and Melzack R (eds). *Textbook of Pain*, 4th edn, churchill livingstone, Edinburgh pp.909–11.

Merskey H and Bogduk N (eds) (1994). *Classification of Chronic Pain: description of chronic pain syndromes and definitions of pain terms.* International Association for the Study of Pain, Seattle.

Mystakidou K, Rosenfeld B, Parpa E, *et al.* (2005). Desire for death near the end of life: The role of depression, anxiety and pain. *General Hospital Psychiatry*, **27**(4), pp.258–62.

National Institute of Clinical Excellence, (2004). NICE guidelines for Depression: management of depression in primary and secondary care. www.nice.org.uk

O'Mahony S, Goulet J, Kornblith A, *et al.* (2005) Desire for hastened death, cancer pain and depression: report of a longitudinal observational study. *Journal of Pain and Symptom Management*, **29**(5), 446–57.

Romano JM and Turner JA (1985). Chronic Pain and Depression: does the evidence support a relationship? *Psychological Bulletin*, **97**(1), 18–34.

Turk DC, Okifuji A, and Scharff L (1995). Chronic pain and depression: role of perceived impact and perceived control in different age cohorts. *Pain*, **61**, 93–101.

Chapter 11

Use of alternative therapies in older people with pain

Panos Barlas

Key points

- Complementary and alternative medicine (CAM) is widely used amongst older adults for the management of a range of painful conditions but its efficacy is largely undemonstrated.
- The evidence for the efficacy of CAM is not in line with its perceived effectiveness perhaps because the underlying mechanisms are unclear, raising the possibility of a non-specific (placebo) response.
- Older adults who use CAM may also have mental health problems and other chronic conditions and it important not to raise unrealistic expectations.
- There is however better evidence for some types of CAM such as acupuncture in the treatment specifically of pain.
- Physicians and other health professionals dealing with older adults should be prepared to offer an unbiased view in terms of best evidence on the likely benefits of CAM for their patients.

11.1 Issues in complementary and alternative medicine

There has been much debate on the subject of terminology used to describe therapies that are outside mainstream medicine but that are frequently used by patients for the treatment of their symptoms. The term 'alternative' implies that they may be used instead of conventional medicine, yet practitioners of these therapies often argue that rather than replace conventional medicine, they complement it. Hence the most acceptable term used for this group of therapies is one that endeavors to include both points of view; 'complementary and alternative medicine' or CAM.

CAM has been defined as 'diagnosis, treatment, and/or prevention which complements mainstream medicine by contributing to a common whole, satisfying a demand not met by orthodoxy, or diversifying the conceptual framework of medicine' (Ernst *et al.* 1995). It may also be said that CAM are practices used for the diagnosis and treatment of disease, not taught widely in medical schools, nor generally available in hospitals (Eisenberg *et al.* 1993).

Population surveys indicate that CAM use is high within the Western world. Surveys indicate that one in three North Americans use some form of CAM and, in the UK, it has been suggested that almost 11% of the population used one or more forms of CAM in 1998, rising to almost 25% by 2002 (Eisenberg *et al.* 1998; Thomas *et al.* 2001).

The most common reasons why patients may choose CAM is because of dissatisfaction with the care offered by conventional medicine, the perception that CAM offers a safer option (than conventional medical treatments), as well as the feeling that CAM therapies treat the patient rather than the disease. In addition, CAM may offer another option when all else fails or, indeed, provide the patient with the feeling of some control over their treatment and allow for the development of a relationship with a therapist who usually has more time and seems more interested than the typical busy NHS physician. Another popular perception is that CAM is 'natural' and therefore 'safe'.

Users as a group are more likely to be female, better educated, and have a higher socioeconomic status, than those who do not use CAM. This probably does not come as a surprise when one takes into account that most of CAM interventions are offered outside conventional publicly funded health-care settings and, therefore, are usually fee-based. Data indicate that the expenditure on CAM practices, modalities, and preparations in the US exceeds government spending in primary health care; similar figures exist for Australian and UK estimated annual costs of CAM.

In contrast to patient views, the medical establishment appears to continue to view CAM with caution. Based on the scientific, biological models of disease and its treatment, it is often difficult for health-care professionals to accept practices that do not seem to make biological sense or that are not based upon scientific evidence of efficacy, effectiveness, and safety (derived from randomized controlled trials) as treatment options for a particular disease. The attitudes of physicians and other health-care professionals towards CAM range from the dismissive and cynical to the integrative, depending on their personal attitudes, experiences of the use of

CAM as well as other demographic factors such as their age (Chen *et al.* 1999; Jump *et al.* 1999; Norheim & Fonnebo, 1998).

Therefore, it is not surprising to hear reports such as that of a patient recovering from cancer, who defined CAM as 'those therapies which, for the past 20 years, I have had to pay for out-of-pocket and never felt comfortable discussing with my physicians' (Eisenberg, 2001).

11.2 Types of CAM

There is an astounding variety of CAM systems and modalities and it is beyond the scope of this chapter to examine each individually. A broad and accepted categorization of CAM has been proposed by the National Centre for Complementary and Alternative Medicine (NCCAM) in the US and can be downloaded from: http://nccam.nih.gov/health/whatiscam/pdf/whatiscam.pdf. Using this classification, CAM modalities can be categorized (Box 11.1).

Of the types mentioned above perhaps the most popular are manipulative and body-based methods and some alternative medical systems such as acupuncture, homeopathy, and self-administered herbal preparations and supplements. In the UK, osteopathy, chiropractic, and acupuncture are reported as the most commonly used forms of CAM. Within the NHS, acupuncture is the most frequent form of CAM offered, typically practised by physiotherapists and, to a lesser extent, by general practitioners and nurses. More than one million acupuncture treatments are given in the NHS annually (Thomas *et al.* 2001).

11.3 Older people and CAM

The high prevalence of painful degenerative conditions such as osteoarthritis and the high use of medications by this patient group seems a likely reason for which older adults may use CAM modalities. Indeed, sufferers from chronic conditions such as arthritis,

Box 11.1 National Centre for Complementary and Alternative Medicine CAM categorization

- Alternative medical systems (i.e., acupuncture, Ayurveda, homeopathy, naturopathy etc.)
- Biologically-based therapies (i.e., chelation therapy, folk medicine, herb use, special diet, or mega-vitamins)
- Manipulative and body-based methods (i.e., chiropractic, osteopathy and massage), and
- Mind–body medicine (i.e., relaxation techniques such as meditation, movement therapies such as yoga, tai-chi, qi-gong and similar healing rituals).

rheumatic disease, diabetes, and cancer are reported to be using CAM more often than the general population. Older people are also likely to be receiving treatment for chronic conditions other than arthritis. Data show that up to 80% of older people with arthritis receive treatment for at least two other chronic conditions (Quandt *et al.* 2005).

A detailed survey in the US suggest that as many as 30% of the population of older adults have used (or are currently using) a CAM modality (Eisenberg *et al.* 1998). Most popular forms of CAM were relaxation techniques, herbal medicines, food supplements, chiropractic, and massage. It is reasonable to assume that this figure is likely to rise, as the population ages and CAM increases in prevalence. More recently, high prevalence of CAM use has been reported amongst older people with mental illness, although, curiously, the modalities used were not always aimed specifically at treating the mental illness and its symptoms (Grzywacz *et al.* 2006). The forms of CAM most frequently used were mind–body medicine, acupuncture, chiropractic, and food supplements.

It has been suggested that older adults use specific CAM modalities for different reasons. Modalities that belong in the 'alternative medical systems' (such as acupuncture, homeopathy etc.), 'manipulative and body-based' therapies (such as massage, osteopathy and chiropractic) and 'biologically-based' therapies (herbal medicine, vitamins etc) are used primarily for treatment of existing conditions and their symptoms, whilst 'mind–body' therapies (relaxation, yoga, tai-chi etc) are used primarily for illness prevention and health promotion (Grzywacz *et al.* 2006).

Studies have shown that certain CAM modalities may be useful in the management of a variety of conditions in older adult populations. As far as pain is concerned the literature has concentrated on the efficacy of modalities with analgesic properties and their effectiveness, predominantly, in the treatment of common musculoskeletal pain. It has been reported that acupuncture is of benefit in the treatment of low back pain (Meng *et al.* 2003), and of knee and hip osteoarthritis (Ezzo *et al.* 2001; Stener Victorin *et al.* 2004) in older adult populations. In particular and in the case of knee osteoarthritis pain, acupuncture has shown analgesic effects for up to a year after treatment (Ezzo *et al.* 2001), whilst acupuncture offered symptomatic relief and functional improvements in patients with hip osteoarthritis for up to six months (Stener-Victorin *et al.* 2004). In both these studies, acupuncture was found to be comparable and in some instances superior to control interventions (e.g. exercise, advice, etc.).

Older adults have a higher risk of experiencing depression and anxiety. It has been shown that it is older patients with affective disorders who are likely to be high users of CAM therapies

(Grzywacz *et al.* 2005; Dello Buono *et al.* 2001). Complementary medicine can offer relief for a range of symptoms other than pain in this group of patients. For example, it has been shown that herbal remedies can help in the management of depression (Grzywacz *et al.* 2005). Specifically St. John's wort (*Hypericum perforatum*) appears to be of benefit for the treatment of mild to moderate depression (Gaster and Holroyd, 2000). Additionally, acupuncture has been shown to help with the treatment of anxiety and insomnia (Suen *et al.* 2003; Spence *et al.* 2004).

CAM use in older adults however, may also have risks to patients. The increasing popularity of manipulative therapies for musculoskeletal pain poses a direct risk for actual injury to the frail and osteoporotic and the use of herbal preparations may interact with other prescription medication (e.g. St John's wort and SSRIs; Ernst *et al.* 2001). The physician should explore these issues by encouraging discussion with the patient and their use of CAM so that patients feel they can discuss all of the available options for the management of their condition.

Whilst there is little conclusive evidence for the usefulness of any particular CAM therapy for the treatment of specific conditions commonly seen in older adults, the general consensus is that CAM interventions may indeed offer viable, relatively safe, and beneficial alternatives to conventional approaches. These benefits may range from pain relief in patients with musculoskeletal pain (for example with acupuncture and massage), to falls prevention (through the practice of yoga and tai-chi). Additionally, anxiety, insomnia, and fatigue may be symptoms for which CAM modalities (for example relaxation, acupuncture, herbal remedies) can offer some relief.

11.4 Conclusions

As can be seen from the above, older adults perceive that they may experience some benefit from the use of CAM modalities. The perceived low risk of adverse reactions associated with the majority of these treatments, the perception of increased involvement in the treatment process, and the empowerment of the patient seem to be attributes of CAM that serve to increase the popularity of CAM amongst older adults and offer further options for relief from common symptoms. Similar to younger populations, older adults who use CAM are usually female, better educated, and are unlikely to be suffering significant disability from chronic somatic disease. However, this patient group appears to have an increased risk of anxiety and depression (Grzywacz *et al.* 2006).

There is public demand for the integration of CAM with conventional medicine and it seems to be an unavoidable and increasing feature of modern medicine. To the extent that the scientific evidence for the efficacy of modalities such as acupuncture, manipulative therapies, and herbal medicine grows, physicians should be increasingly willing to consider these modalities as additional options for the care of their patients. For example, most primary health-care facilities and NHS hospitals are now offering acupuncture and manipulation, and an increasing number of general practitioners and physiotherapists are now trained in these practices. Medical schools are increasingly offering courses on homeopathy, acupuncture, and other forms of CAM at undergraduate level. Nonetheless there remains an obligation to evaluate treatment carefully and be prepared to move from uncritical acceptance of CAM simply because it is 'an alternative' and to develop a much sharper focus on what works for whom.

Patient demand for solutions to their health-care problems, other than pharmacological or surgical options, and an increasing volume of research suggesting the benefits of some forms of CAM interventions, dictate the need for practitioners to be informed about CAM interventions and their potential benefits and risks. Health-care professionals should talk to their patients and encourage disclosure and discussion of the use of alternative practices. This will ensure that patients feel more involved in the management of their illness and allow for appropriate advice can be given.

References

Chen *et al.* (1999). Differences between familiy physicians and patients in their knowledge and attitudes regarding traditional Chinese medicine. *Int Med*, **2**, 45–55.

Dello Buono M, *et al.* (2001). Alternative medicine in a sample of 655 community-dwelling elderly. *J Psychosom Res*, **50**, 147–54.

Ezzo J, *et al.* (2001). Acupuncture for osteoarthritis of the knee: a systematic review. *Arthr Rheum*, **44**, 819–25.

Eisenberg DM, *et al.* (1993). Unconventional medicine in the United States: prevalence, costs and patterns of use. *N Engl J Med*, **328**, 246–52.

Eisenberg DM, *et al.* (1998). Trends in alternative medicine use in the United States, 1990–1997: results of a follow-up national survey. *JAMA*, **280**, 1569–75.

Eisenberg D, (2001) Complementary and alternative medicine use in the United States: Epidemiology and Trends 1990–2000. In Ernst E (ed). *The desktop guide to complementary and alternative medicine*. Mosby, London. pp.374–87.

Ernst E *et al.* (1995). Complementary medicine- a definition. *Br J Gen Pract*, **309**,107–11.

Ernst E, (ed) (2001). *The desktop guide to complementary and alternative medicine*. Mosby: London.

Gaster B, and Holroyd J (2000). St. John's wort for depression: a systematic review. *Arch Intern Med*, **160**, 152–6.

Grzywacz JG, *et al.* (2005). Age, race and ethnicity in the use of complementary and alternative medicine for health self-management. *J Aging Health,* **17**, 547–72.

Grzywacz JG, *et al.* (2006). Older adults' use of complementary and alternative medicine for mental health: Findings from the 2002 National Health Interview Survey. *J Alt Comp Med,* **12**(5), 467–73.

Jump J, *et al.* (1999). Physician's attitudes toward complementary and alternative Medicine. *Int Med*, **1**, 149–53.

Meng CF, *et al.* (2003). Acupuncture for chronic low back pain in older patients: a randomized controlled trial. Rheumatology, **42**, 1–10.

Norheim AJ and Fonnebo V (1998). Doctors' attitudes to acupuncture- a Norwegian study. *Soc Sci Med*, **47**(4), 519–23.

Quandt SA, *et al.* (2005). Use of complementary and alternative medicine by persons with arthritis: the results of the National Health Interview Survey. *Arthr Rheum*, **53**, 748–55.

Spence DW, *et al.* (2004). Acupuncture increases nocturnal melatonin secretion and reduces insomnia and anxiety: a preliminary report. *J Neuropsychiatry Clin Neurosci*, **16**, 19–28.

Stener-Victorin E et *al.* (2004). Comparison between electro-acupuncture and hydrotherapy, both in combination with patient education and patient education alone, on the symptomatic treatment of osteoarthritis of the hip. *Clin J Pain*, **20**, 179–85.

Suen LKP, *et al.* (2003). The long-term effects of auricular therapy using magnetic pearls on elderly with insomnia. *Comp Ther Med*, **11**, 85–92.

Thomas K, *et al.* (2001). Use and expenditure on complementary medicine in England: a population based survey. *Comp Ther Med*, **9**, 2–11.

Chapter 12

Occupational therapy and physiotherapy

Bhanu Ramaswamy, Jill Chanter, and Claire Craig

Key points

- Occupational and physiotherapists work to enable the older person in pain to achieve maximum independence and quality of life.
- Prompt assessment minimizes the risk of pain leading to inactivity and body deconditioning.
- Overall, the occupational therapist elicits the meaning of pain to the individual and its impact on their role and sense of self.
- In general, the physiotherapist focuses on recovery of function, reduction and prevention of pain from condition or age-related musculo-skeletal changes.
- Therapists complement multidisciplinary team interventions by addressing barriers that may prevent optimal functioning of older people in pain. This assists the person to cope and/or recover from the pain.

12.1 Introduction

Occupational therapists (OTs) and physiotherapists work alongside older people in a range of hospital and community settings. They assess the impact of illness and disability on physical, psychological, and social functions and, through a structured programme of activity, work with the individual to achieve maximum independence and quality of life. Whilst the end goals for each profession may be similar, the rationale of the clinical decision making process differs.

This chapter provides a general overview of the main approaches utilized by the two therapies in the management of older people where pain either presents as the primary problem, or is secondary to the condition being treated. Pain is a complex process, and the aim of this chapter will be to outline the principles of intervention relevant to acute, chronic, and oncological pain in older people.

Full and timely assessment from the therapies is of paramount importance to prevent pain leading to the spiral of inactivity and reduced quality of life (Figure 12.1).

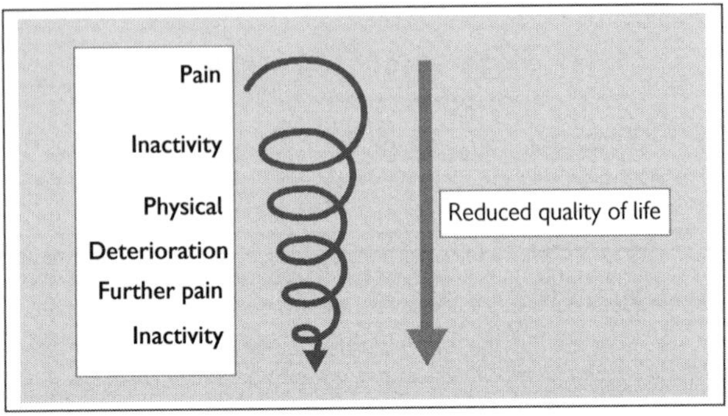

Figure 12.1 The spiral of pain related inactivity and reduced quality of life. An illustration of the inter-relationship between pain and inactivity (Craig 2006, based on Strong, 2002).

12.2 Occupational therapy and pain in older people

12.2.1 Why refer to occupational therapy?

OT focuses on the physical, emotional and social effects of illness and disability with the aim of improving coping strategies in the individual's ability to carry out the activities that they need or choose to do in their daily lives (COT 2006).

The impact of pain on individual function, activity, and relationships can be neglected or dismissed as an inevitable part of ageing and consequently under-treated (Cavalieri 2002). However, when combined with ageing processes it can lead to a swift decline in mobility and function in older people. Disengagement from meaningful activities, from valued roles and routines may result in low mood and poor self-esteem (Craig & Mountain, 2006).

Such problems are often intensified because the domains of pain i.e. sensory-discriminative, cognitive-evaluative, and motivational-affective, are interactive dimensions. These contribute to an individual's sense of self. For older people, their sense of self is challenged when not equipped to effectively manage their pain further compromising their independence and quality of life (Harris *et al.* 2003).

12.2.2 **When to refer to occupational therapy**

Early referral to specialist OT services minimizes the risk of loss of function and identity where the older person is locked into a negative spiral. It provides an alternative to the structural, pathological medical model.

OT referral should be triggered when pain results in problems experienced whilst performing activities of daily living, personal (washing, dressing, transferring from bed chair or bath) domestic (cooking, shopping, cleaning) and social (roles, relationships and networks).

12.2.3 **Occupational therapy assessment**

In order to gain a full picture of how pain is impacting/encroaching on the older person's life, OTs utilize a number of tools to build a holistic picture (Table 12.1).

Table 12.1 Occupational therapy assessment tools

Assessment of function	Activities of daily living checklist, observation, home assessment of the person undertaking daily tasks, Extended Barthel Index
Roles and routines	Role checklist (establishing valued roles and routines). Occupational performance history interview
Quality of life	Short Form health survey (SF-36). Self-report measure of health-related quality of life
Mood	Geriatric depression scale, Beck's Depression Inventory

Underpinning all assessment is the ability to elicit the meaning that pain has for the individual. For example, fundamental to independence is the apparently straightforward activity of getting out of a chair. The individual's description of their experience can provide valuable information that indicates the source of the problem (Box 12.1).

Box 12.1 The relationship of activity to the dimensions of pain

'The pain in my back increases when I get out of a chair (sensory discriminative), I might make my pain even worse (cognitive-evaluative) so I won't bother to try and then I get depressed (motivational-affective)'.

Alternatively: 'The pain in my back increases when I get out of my chair, I will have to try harder but however determined I am the pain gets worse and I get fustrated'.

These descriptions illustrate how pain is shaped by the context in which it is experienced and understood in terms of damage and consequences. This cognitive-evaluative component interacts with the sensory-discriminative establishing whether the experience fits with the individual's expectation, intensity, and location of pain. The degree of correlation may then influence the motivational-affective response and behaviour.

12.2.4 Intervention by occupational therapists

By establishing the individual's experience of the pain, the OT can then address issues raised. The process requires education of both the person and their family about the changing nature of pain at the acute, chronic, or terminal stages. This promotes engagement with appropriate strategies (Table 12.2).

Table 12.2 Educational strategies to manage pain
Clarification of the meaning of pain for the individual and language used by health professionals in explaining the causes of pain, 'wear and tear'; 'crumbling spine'; 'degenerative joints' to minimize iatrogenesis.
Exploration of more subtle issues about the inevitability of pain in the elderly, the expectation of stoicism, fear of immobility and dependence.
Facilitation of the transition from the cognitions of 'hurt equals harm', 'beat the pain', 'there must be a cure for this pain', to those of managing the pain and adopting effective coping strategies.
Utillization of adaptive pain coping strategies to facilitate resumption of roles and activities by a process of adjustment and acceptance (MC cracken & Eccleston 2005).

The OT then works collaboratively to set goals that the individual can work towards. To achieve these goals the therapist may help the person to develop a problem solving approach to gain understanding of factors that make the pain worse during activity and explore strategies to ease or lessen the pain, (Box 12.2). Impaired cognition due to such conditions as dementia or confusion (see Chapter 3), may become barriers to this type of intervention, and alternative strategies may need to be sought.

Box 12.2 Influences on pain

Factors that make the pain worse during activity:	Strategies that may ease the pain:
• Holding breath • Increased muscle tension • Postural changes • Inefficient use of body mechanics	• Heat • Deep breathing • Distraction • Effective use of body mechanics • Joint protection • Energy conservation • Activities that the person finds restorative or relaxing • Specific techniques to promote relaxation

Where appropriate the OT may also provide appropriate aids and adaptations or orthoses to optimize function.

By focusing on engaging the individual with active management strategies the occupational therapist is able to complement multidisciplinary team interventions by addressing barriers that may prevent optimal application.

12.3 Physiotherapy and pain in older people

12.3.1 Introduction

Physiotherapy uses physical approaches to promote, maintain, and restore physical, psychological and social well-being whilst accounting for a person's health status (CSP, 2002). Whilst physiotherapists' particular skills lie in the assessment and treatment of mechanical functioning, it is especially important to recognize the impact of all domains when working with older people (Shacklock, 1999).

12.3.2 When to refer to a physiotherapist

Referral to physiotherapy would be to assist recovery of function for alleviation of pain experienced by an older person to allow continued participation in their chosen lifestyle.

As soon as new pain or altering functional ability (and loss of independence) is identified, a referral should be made. Physiotherapy is most effective in treating new or exacerbative pain processes of known musculo-skeletal origin e.g. arthritis, or for unassessed chronic pain conditions.

It is unacceptable to assume that just because a person is old they should 'expect' to experience pain. It is also unethical to expect acceptance of pain without a treatment offer from medical diagnoses where pain will be a known symptom e.g. in certain cancers.

Assessment and the subsequent intervention should not be delayed as the complex nature of ageing on the bio-psychosocial aspects of the older person's life may mean the difference of continued ability to live independently at home (plus additional support if necessary) versus unnecessary admission to secondary care for preventable diagnoses such as '*acopia*' and '*gone off legs*' (McCaffery & Pasero, 1999).

12.3.3 What to understand about referral to physiotherapy for pain management in older people

As with other professions, it is imperative that the referring individual recognizes that there are specialisms within physiotherapy with capacity to deal with pain differently. In general it is appropriate to refer to a specialist as explained in Box 12.3.

Clinical evidence for physiotherapy intervention for pain in the older population is growing (Hertling & Kessler, 2006). Much practice however is also based on clinical reasoning from trials on younger populations to advise on treatments for the older generation, and it must also be noted that the older literature does not adhere to the robust methodology expected of today's studies.

Box 12.3 Physiotherapy specialisms dealing with pain in older people

- 'Out-patient' type physiotherapy for assessment and management of isolated areas of presenting pain, especially for dysfunction of mechanical, musculo-skeletal origin.
- 'Chronic pain team' specialist physiotherapy (with access to psychological support) for longer-term complex and intractable pain when other avenues have been tried and surgical intervention is undesirable.
- Older person rehabilitation specialists e.g. Community Rehabilitation or Intermediate Care team physiotherapist, if the older person requires a more holistic pain-coping approach inclusive of lifestyle issues, enabling social service support and fear avoidance strategies. These physiotherapists often provide longer-term, initially more concentrated intervention, especially for those with general debilitative conditions.
- Physiotherapists specialising in oncology for older people with pain from lymphoedema or active cancerous pathology.

12.3.4 Assessment by physiotherapists

Assessment of pain includes subjective and objective assessments leading to a clear clinical diagnosis.

12.3.4.1 *Subjective*

Appropriate questioning allows the therapist to examine the pain and its effect on the older person, once it has been established why they have presented and what their expectation is from physiotherapy. The subjective examination also ensures the physiotherapist has acquired the information enabling clinical decisions to be made regarding the subsequent physical assessment. See Box 12.4.

Box 12.4 Subjective assessment of an older person's pain

Subjective assessments should always include:

- History of presenting condition
- Past medical history
- Current medications being taken, including over the counter drugs and herbal remedies
- Social history, inclusive of lifestyle alterations due to pain
- Location and quality of pain
- Pain behaviour including aggravating and easing factors, previous experience of pain and how they dealt with it
- Impact on functional ability
- Barriers to the patient's ability to deal with the pain

Location of pain

Reported pain may be misleading with older people. It might be:

- At the site of injury.
- Referred e.g. sciatic pain down a leg.
- Secondary to the original cause. For example, following a fall with jarring to the shoulder, recovery of the initial insult occurs, but there may be altered limb functioning subsequent to the initial protective response. The changes within the shoulder joint complex or mistiming of muscle action patterns will result in pain on certain movements.

Quality of pain

- More difficult to use for clinical diagnosis when described by older people.
- Acute pain from obvious causes e.g. fracture, surgery, pneumonia is usually more accurately described.
- As sensory feedback diminishes with age, interpretation and perception of 'general' pain is altered; it may be summarized as 'soreness' or 'aching'.
- This might affect the therapist's ability to distinguish between origins of pain e.g. neural, mechanical especially as in many cases, it may be of a combined source e.g. aggravated sciatica from a recent injurious fall and hence both nociceptive and neuropathic in nature (Herman & Scudds 1995).
- There is also poor correlation between presenting pain and radiological tests.

Aggravating and easing factors

- Includes questioning of the behaviour and pattern of the presentation of pain as well as the speed in which pain appears and can be eased.
- In older people, less obvious reasons might cause pain e.g. a wheelchair used for prolonged sitting with poor pelvic and back support, history of chronic constipation.
- Persistence of pain, especially in the lower back, may occur from a myriad of mechanisms (Cavanaugh, 1995). Identification of the position where the pain is eased may be an indication to the therapist of when the structure at fault is not under stress, and what interventions might be appropriate.

Impact of pain on functional ability

- The nature of pain is personal as is the character, attitude and experience of the person in pain. A stoical person will continue to mobilise despite their pain, whilst someone with the same pathology plus low pain tolerance and mood may not be able to get out of bed.

Barriers to the patient's ability to deal with the pain

These are often multi-factorial in older people and include a combination of issues as explored in Box 12.5.

Box 12.5 Barriers to dealing successfully with pain

- Self-ageist attitudes, expecting pain as part of the ageing process.
- Well established beliefs and 'acceptances' about pain.
- Understanding of pain causing conditions, especially limited in those with limited attention or cognitive impairment (see Chapter 3).
- Mental state to deal effectively with the longer-term commitments to alleviation of pain if depressed or anxious.
- Expectations of interventions, whether from past experience or hearsay.
- Whether the pain element has become part of a dynamic within a relationship with significant others (Harris *et al.* 2003).
- Other pathology compounding the pain or altering things such as pharmacokinetics, and hence response to analgesia.

12.3.4.2 ***Objective***

The objective assessment confirms the subjective history allowing a clinical diagnosis that may be different to the 'label' ascribed the person on referral to be made. It also enables the practitioner to identify 'red flags' that would require referral on for further investigation.

It is important to consider the setting(s) of the assessment when dealing with older people with longer-term pain. An older person who attends an 'OA knee' class may show improvement in objective markers used by the physiotherapist but this does not indicate their coping ability at home. If under-reporting of pain is suspected, a referral to domiciliary physiotherapy allows assessment of the person's home. Such things like untidiness or self-neglect will highlight the impact and limitations in activities caused by the pain more than a measure of increased walking distance or joint range in a physiotherapy department.

The objective assessment itself includes specific joint, nerve, and muscle tests to assess function and quality of these structures. It may recreate the pain or elicit a relevant sign that may indicate a cause of pain allowing a clinical diagnosis. In frail older people, it is especially important to assess the person's functional ability and pain responses to flexibility, strength, power, and endurance testing, plus the impact of pain on balance, co-ordination, and function, as these last three are the physical manifestations that affect independence (Gurnalik *et al.* 2001).

12.3.5 **Intervention by physiotherapy**

Physiotherapy offers a mainly non-pharmacological and often non-invasive solution to pain control although intervention may be in conjunction with analgesics. In addition to providing an explanation about the pain in terms of body biomechanics and causes of the person's pain, their perception and its impact on their life (Moseley 2006), physiotherapy might also include a combination of approaches. If intervention cannot eliminate the pain, it can at least diminish its effects to a level more acceptable to the sufferer (Box 12.6).

Box 12.6 Main pain relieving techniques used with older people

- Education
- Thermotherapy such as ice/heat
- Exercise
- Manual therapy
- Massage
- Assessment for supportive or assistive devices to regain lost mobility
- Some electrotherapy e.g. transcutaneous electrical nerve stimulation (TENS), electroacupuncture
- Taping
- Invasive techniques such as injections or acupuncture.

The evidence base for this generic section is too large to be included in full; the reader is advised to seek information though the major databases, especially the Cochrane and the Physiotherapy Evidence Databases (PEDro) from where substantiation can be acquired.

12.3.5.1 *Education on pain management*

- Correct understanding of the reason for the pain followed by provision of information and support to address it is vital.
- It allows a person to cope/manage their pain (Moseley 2006, 2003).
- With older people, verbal information should be supplemented with written information and instructions (user-friendly publications are available from many different disease specific voluntary agencies and charities).
- Dealing with pain-related fear must be undertaken a soon as possible to prevent the deterioration of mobility and its consequences (Cook *et al.* 2006).

12.3.5.2 ***Thermotherapy: heat***

- Heat is a short-term pain relieving modality enjoyed by many older people although evidence is limited as to its clinical effectiveness due to the limitations of markers and qualitative measurement supporting its use.
- It is recommended as an adjunct to further manual intervention (Önes *et al.* 2006) due to effect of enhancing the flexibility of the underlying tissues.

12.3.5.3 ***Ice***

- Ice is not always a welcome modality with older people unless the joint is hot and swollen; they feel the cold more acutely than heat. It is a useful adjunct to intervention, especially if it relieves pain and oedema.
- The condition of thinner, more frail skin must be assessed before ice is used, and the length of time for which it is applied be more closely monitored.

12.3.5.4 ***Exercise***

- Exercise is essential to deal with chronic pain conditions and is the mainstay of physiotherapy interventions for older people with pain (Morris & Schoo, 2004).
- Supportive networks, whether through a church, family, friends, referral to the other multidisciplinary team members etc. are an important aspect to continued ability to maintain function or the ability to carry on with a prescribed programme of exercise (Roddy *et al.* 2005) to minimize, prevent the recurrence of injury and pain and generally ensure the longer term benefits (Wilder *et al.* 2006).

12.3.5.5 ***Acute soft tissue pain management***

- Management of soft tissue (musculoskeletal) during the first 72 hours injury using protection, rest, ice, compression, and elevation (PRICE) (Kerr *et al.* 2002) does not differ with older people.
- The response to the varying interventions require close monitoring, e.g. compression may not be appropriate for someone with distal oedema that may worsen and lead to vascular compromize; the use of ice will need extra monitoring; elevated positions may need to be modified if underlying structures are not sufficiently flexible.

12.3.5.6 ***Assessment for supportive or assistive devices to regain lost mobility***

- Pain might be alleviated through the use of orthotic devices to balance structural anomalies e.g. shoe raises for leg-length discrepancies, knee braces to provide proprioceptive input to the quadriceps for an arthritic knee that buckles, progression from sticks to crutches or a frame to spread the load from a painful weight bearing joint.

12.3.5.7 ***Massage and specific soft tissue mobilization***

- Older people respond well to massage and specific soft tissue mobilization due to the combined effect on the body and mind.
- Therapeutically it enhances blood flow and analgesic effects but the physiotherapist also gains much from the tactile information gained from palpation of soft tissue, and its response to the treatment.
- It can indicate the state of compliance of the tissue and joints in terms of their 'readiness' to be facilitated into functional movement, or if there is pain-induced inhibition to activity. The former is especially the case with people who have neurological deficits causing limbs to be held in fixed positions for a long period, and the latter seen in people with longer-term back pain of pain from arthritic joints (Hides *et al.* 1996).

12.3.5.8 ***Manual therapies***

- Specific modalities such as Mackenzie, Maitland etc., may be useful tools in providing pain relief from mechanical causes of pain in older people due to the dampening effect to pain responses the interventions have on the central nervous system.
- The practitioner must be aware of other pathologies that might adversely affect the treatment such as osteoporosis.
- A more eclectic approach of interventions is suggested, and always to be followed by active treatment e.g. exercises, to maintain the effects of these more passive modalities.
- With longer-term management/prevention of recurrence of pain, this allows the person more independence and responsibility for management of their own condition, as many older people are used to a more medical model of 'being made better' by the practitioner.

12.3.5.9 ***Electrotherapy***

- Electrotherapy modalities such as electromagnetic energy and ultrasound (US) have become less popular choices when treating pain in older people due to the increasing evidence of lack of effect.
- TENS is an electrotherapy modality still in use. It has been suggested that therapeutic benefits are better from the higher price range TENS machine models.
- The person with pain is in control of the machine in terms of setting adjustment, frequency of use, and duration, although pain may not last longer than the duration it is applied.
- The less supple older person can however find the settings fiddly, or be unable to access the necessary body part to apply the electrodes, so availability of support should be ascertained before this modality is employed.
- The machine may also be out of the price range of the older person if they are expected to purchase one.

12.3.5.10 ***Acupuncture***

- A skin-invasive pain relief technique, usually well tolerated by older people with increasing evidence of its efficacy in managing pain (Ezzo *et al.* 2000; Longworth, 2006).

12.4 Outcome measures used by occupational therapists and physiotherapists

Occupational and physiotherapists involved with older people who present with pain work to achieve maximum independence and quality of life through various interventions. Whilst a simple measure of efficacy might be the reduction in pain though the use of a visual analogue scale, the impact/outcome of interventions should also be measured in terms of the ability of the recipient to execute an activity, as well the capacity to function in their chosen environment (Üstün *et al.* 2003) whether the pain has been alleviated, or whether the person has been taught to cope with it (Box 12.7).

A wide range of outcome measures exist depending on what the therapist (or team) is trying to measure and there is a growing evidence base for use of appropriately selected measures reflecting the bio-psycho-social manifestation of pain on the individual's quality of life (Bowling, 1995).

Box 12.7 Measurement of intervention

Measurement is encompassed through some of the following areas:

- Optimization of independence through adaptation or support
- Promotion of increased activity
- Increased self-efficacy.
- Resumption of valued roles
- Reported feelings of well-being
- Reported decrease in pain levels, although it is important to relate this to any of the above.

12.5 Conclusions

This chapter has outlined the key roles that OT and physiotherapy can play in the management of pain in older people. In understanding the relationship between activity and pain in the older person therapists are able to complement multi disciplinary team interventions and address barriers that may prevent the individuals' optimal functioning.

References

Bowling A (1995). *Measuring disease*. Open University Press, Buckingham.

Cavalieri TA (2002). Pain management in the elderly. *Journal of the American Osteopathic Association,* **102** (9), 481–5.

Cavanaugh JM (1995). Neural mechanisms of lumbar pain. *Spine*, **20**(16), 1804–09.

Chartered Society of Physiotherapy (2002). *Curriculum Framework.* London, CSP.

Cochrane database, Available at: http://www.nelh.nhs.uk/cochrane.asp

College of Occupation Therapists (2006). *Definitions and Core Skills for Occupational Therapy*. COT/BAOT Briefings 23. Available at: http://www.cot.org.uk/members/publications/free/briefings/pdf/23Definitions&CoreSkills.pdf. Accessed 23.06.06.

Cook A, Brawer P, and Vowels K (2006). The fear-avoidance model of chronic pain: Validation and age analysis using structural equation modelling. *Pain,* **121**, 195–206.

Craig C and Mountain G (in press). *Lifestyle matters: An occupational approach to healthy ageing*. Speechmark, Bicester.

Ezzo J, Berman B, Hadhazy VA, *et al.* (2000). Is acupuncture effective for the treatment of chronic pain? A systematic review. *Pain,* **86**(3), 217–25.

Gurnalik J, Ferruci L, Balfour J, *et al.* (2001). Progressive versus catastrophic loss of the ability to walk: Implications for the prevention of mobility loss. *J American Geriatric Society*, **49**, 1463–70.

Harris S, Morley S, and Barton S (2003). Role loss and emotional adjustment in chronic pain, *Pain*, **105**, 363–70.

Herman E and Scudds R (1995). *Pain.* In Pickles B, Compton A, Cott C, *et al.* (eds). *Physiotherapy with older people*. WB Saunders, London.

Hertling D and Kessler R (2006). *Management of common musculoskeletal disorders: Physical therapy principles and methods. Fourth edition.* Lippincott Williams and Wilkins, Philadelphia.

Hides J, Richardson C, and Jull G (1996). Multifidus muscle recovery is not automatic after resolution of acute, first-episode low back pain. *Spine*, **21**(23), 2763–69.

Kerr K, Booth L, Daley L, *et al.* (2002). *Guidelines for the management of soft tissue injury during the first 72 hours.* ACPSM, CSP, London.

Longworth W (2006). Acupuncture in palliative care. *J Acupuncture Association of Chartered Physiotherapists;* January, 26–30.

McCaffery M and Pasero C (1999). *Pain: Clinical Manual. Second edition.* Mosby, St. Louis MO.

McCracken L and Eccleston C. (2005). A Comparison of the relative utility of coping and acceptance-based measures in a sample of chronic pain sufferers. *European Journal of Pain,* **10**, 23–29.

Morris M and Schoo A (eds) (2004). *Optimising exercise and physical activity in older people.* Butterworth-Heinemann, Edinburgh.

Moseley L (2006). Explain pain and getting the message to patients. *In Touch (Summer issue)*; **115**; 12–17.

Moseley L (2003). Unravelling the barriers to reconceptualization of the problem in chronic pain: the actual and perceived ability of patients and healthcare professionals to understand neurophysiology. *The Journal of Pain*, **4**(4), 184–9.

Önes K, Tetic S, Tetik C, Önes N (2006). The effects of heat on osteoarthritis of the knee. *The Pain Clinic*, **18**(1), 67–75.

Physiotherapy Evidence Databases (PEDro) database, Available at: http://www.pedro.fhs.usyd.edu.au/index.html.

Roddy E, Zhang W, and Doherty M (2005). Evidence-based recommendations for the role of exercise in the management of osteoarthritis of the hip and Knee – the MOVE consensus. *Rheumatology (Oxford)*, **44**(1), 67–73.

Shacklock MO (1999). Central pain mechanisms: A new horizon in manual therapy. *Australian Journal of Physiotherapy*, **45**, 83–92.

Strong J (2002). Lifestyle management. In Strong, Unruh AM, Wright A, *et al.* (eds) *Pain: a textbook for therapists*. Churchill Livingstone, London.

Üstün TB, Chatterji S, Bickenbach J, *et al.* (2003). The international classification of functioning, disability and health: A new tool for understanding disability and health. *Disability and Rehabilitation*; **25**(11–12), 565–71.

Wilder F, Barrett J, and Farina E (2006). Exercise and osteoarthritis: Are we stopping too early? Findings from the Clearwater Exercise Study. *Journal of Aging and Physical Activity*, **14**, 169–80.

Chapter 13

Palliative care, cancer care, and end of life

Lisa Beeston

Key points

- Annually in the United Kingdom 200,000 people develop cancer. The likelihood of developing cancer increases as we age.
- Pain related to cancer is a complex phenomenon which encompasses physical, social, psychological, and spiritual aspects of care—all of these have to be taken into account when caring for a person in pain.
- Despite the fact that pain control in people with cancer is a significant problem, it can be managed effectively in the majority of cases, particularly when recommended guidelines are incorporated into practice.
- The traditional focus for palliative care has been cancer care within the hospice setting. There is a need to recognize that although cancer care, palliative care, and end-of-life care are related, the principles of good palliative care can be transferred to non hospice settings.

13.1 Introduction

In many ways a chapter which is entitled 'palliative care, cancer and end of life' can be seen to be problematic; not everyone who has cancer will die from the disease, and not everyone who needs access to good palliative care will have cancer. However, the focus for this chapter will be cancer related pain in older people, and care relating to issues at the end of life, bearing in mind that the principles of good palliative care and pain management can be transferred to non cancer settings.

Annually in the UK 200,000 people are diagnosed with cancer, and approximately 120,000 people die from the disease (Department of Health, 2000). More than a third of cancers are diagnosed in people who are over 75 years of age, and the proportion of the United Kingdom population who are this age and over is set to increase from around 7% to nearly 11% in the next 50 years (Turner *et al.* 1999). In developed countries approximately 60% of cancer patients are 65 years and over (Jovecevic–Bekic 2002).

One of the problems which has become apparent over the last few years is that we are not always clear about the best way to investigate and treat older people with cancer because many of the clinical treatment trials which have taken place have arbitrary upper age limits, and there is substantial under representation of patients who are 65 years and older within these trials (Turner *et al.* 1999).

13.1.1 **Pain related to cancer**

Pain is one of the most common and probably most feared symptoms of advanced cancer and the prevalence of chronic pain in patients with advanced cancer is 70–90 % (Portenoy *et al.* 1994). Because pain is a complex phenomenon with a variety of physical and non-physical factors contributing to how that pain is perceived, it is important to ensure that pain relief encompasses physical, psychological, social and spiritual aspects of care (Fallon *et al.* 2006). For example, if you or I have abdominal pain we may put it down to a temporary and reversible cause. On the other hand, a patient who has had a previous diagnosis of ovarian cancer might perceive a similar pain to be more intense, severe, serious and life threatening. This will affect the meaning of the pain and perhaps how the person copes with it. In a review of the literature, Sutton *et al.* (2002) point out that psychological factors can influence a patient's experience of pain and they suggest that the intensity of pain experienced by patients with advanced cancer is related to their psychological and emotional distress since patients with higher levels of pain are more likely to report mood disturbance and negative emotional states. However, it is not certain if it is the pain which is increasing the psychological and emotional distress or vice versa. In addition to the pharmacological strategies outlined below, psychological and social support are important aspects of care which we need to incorporate into our practice.

Pain control in people with cancer remains a significant problem even though it can be managed effectively in up to 90 per cent of patients with relatively simple drug therapies (Agency for Health Care Policy and Research 1994). Cleary and Carbone (2000) point out that older patients are less likely than younger patients to receive proper pain management. In a systematic assessment of pain in older patients with cancer Bernabei *et al.* (1999) discovered that patients aged 85 years and older were less likely to receive morphine or other strong opiates than those aged 65–74 years. More than a quarter of patients in daily pain included in their large study did not receive any analgesic agent. This is despite the recognition of the widespread under treatment of cancer pain which led to the publication of the World Health Organization (WHO, 1990) recommended guidelines for pain relief in cancer which consists of a three step ladder (see Figure 13.1).

Figure 13.1 The World Health Organization's 3-Step pain relief ladder (WHO, 1990)

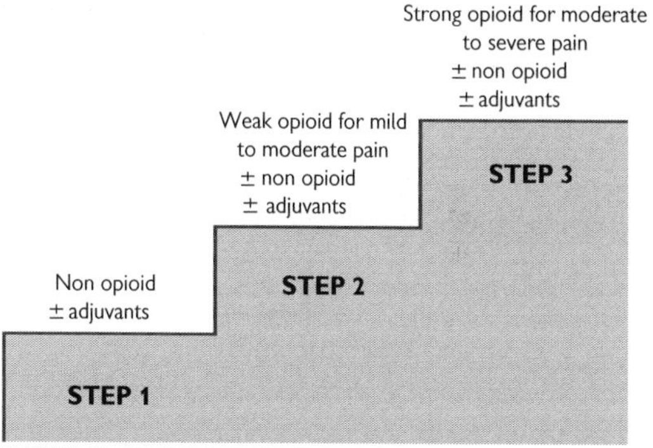

Evaluations of the effectiveness of the WHO recommendations suggest that they provide an effective basis for the treatment of pain in advanced cancer (Agency for Health Care Policy and Research, 1994, Zech *et al.* 1995). The recommendation is that if pain occurs then there should be prompt treatment guided by the following principles (Boxes 13.1–4) of analgesic use (adapted from Twycross, 1997).

Box 13.1 Principles of analgesic use

By the mouth

The oral route is the preferred route of administration. This is because regular injections can tie the patient to a second person and can limit the control the patient has over their own medication. Indications for injections include intractable vomiting, an inability to swallow, coma, poor absorption, or an aversion to oral medication. Recent trials with transdermal fentanyl have shown it to be highly effective and it may be the opiate of choice in patients who have side effects such as nausea, drowsiness and constipation from morphine (Ahmedazi & Brooks, 1997). The transdermal approach may also be beneficial if patients have difficulty remembering to take their medication.

Box 13.2 Principles of analgesic use

By the clock

Because cancer pain tends to be chronic in nature, the pain is likely to return if adequate analgesics are not administered on a regular basis. This means that drugs should be given 'by the clock'—that is for example every 4 hours, depending upon the pharmacological activity of the prescribed drug. It is also necessary to ensure that adequate breakthrough doses of appropriate analgesia are also prescribed if needed.

Box 13.3 Principles of analgesic use

By the ladder

Using the WHO 3-step analgesic ladder (Figure 13.1) provides a means for titrating analgesics against the amount of pain a person is experiencing. If a drug fails to relieve pain then the recommendation is to move up the ladder and not laterally to drugs in the same group. However, a word of caution is necessary here since if the dose of an opiate has been increased by 50% with no improvement in symptoms and the patient is experiencing side effects from the drug then it might not be an opiate responsive pain and further assessment will be necessary.

Box 13.4 Principles of analgesic use

Individual treatment and supervision

It is essential that the response to treatment is monitored closely to ensure that treatment effects are maximized and side effects minimized. Initial and ongoing assessment of a person's pain is crucial in order to ensure that the type of pain (somatic/nociceptive, visceral, or neuropathic) and its intensity is accurately diagnosed and treated. Careful assessment is the key to effective management (Kaye, 1999). In patients with more than one pain, each pain should be re-evaluated (Twycross, 1997). A range of pharmacological interventions might be necessary bearing in mind that visceral or soft tissue pain tends to respond well to morphine. Bone pain may respond well to non steroidal anti inflammatory drugs (NSAIDs), and nerve pain may require the use one or more secondary analgesics such as Tricyclic antidepressants and/or anticonvulsants (i.e. drugs not marketed primarily as analgesics but of value in relieving nerve pain) and steroids, depending upon the type of nerve pain. The concept of nerve pain in cancer is explored separately below.

Part of the strategy for individual (pharmacological) treatment for cancer pain is the recognition that pain is complex, may have a variety of causes and, that a range of factors need to be taken into account when commencing a person on a new analgesic. Kaye (1999) discusses some of these complex issues in the flow charts (Figures 13.2 and 13.3).

Figure 13.2 Pain control

Question	Answer	Action
Is it very **severe** (e.g. seriously disturbing sleep)?	Yes	**Severe pain** is a medical emergency—consider admission.
(No ↓) Is the pain due to **cancer**?	No	**Medical and surgical pains** can still occur (e.g. angina, peptic ulcer, renal colic, carpal tunnel).
(Yes ↓) Is it a new **continuous** aching pain?	Yes	**Visceral or soft tissue pains** nearly always respond to opioids.
(No ↓) Is it **recurrent** continuous aching pain, despite opioids?	Yes	**Cellulitis** can do this—especially in head and neck tumours • Broad spectrum antibiotic
(No ↓) Is it worse on the **slightest movement**?	Yes	**Fracture** • X-ray • Arrange internal fixation wherever possible
(No ↓) Is it related to general **movement** or weight-bearing	Yes	**Bone pain** • Confirm metastases by bone scan ± X-ray • Palliative RT • NSAIDs
(No ↓) Is it related to **breathing**?	Yes	**Pleuritic pain** consider: • chest infection • pulmonary embolus • fractured rib • nerve root (bilateral) from spinal disease
(No ↓) Is it **burning or stabbing**?	Yes	**Nerve pain** • Severe, difficult to control • Partial response to opioids • Tricyclics help 40% • Anticonvulsants help 30% • Steroids help a few
(No ↓) Is it **colicky** (coming and going every few minutes) and **abdominal**?	Yes	**Abdominal colic** • Exclude constipation • Buscopan (oral or SC) • Remember gallstones (U/S scan)
(No ↓) Is it **colicky** in the **back** or side?	Yes	**Renal or ureteric** • IM diclofenac • Ureteric stent? • Nephrostomy?
(No ↓) Is it **colicky** and **suprapubic**?	Yes	**Bladder spasm** • Diclofenac 75mg IM • Buscopan SC 80mg/24h • Oxybutinin 5mg TID • Instill local anaesthetic?
(No ↓) Is it **spasm** in the back passage?	Yes	**Tenesmus** • Exclude constipation • NSAIDs • Colifoam enemas • Transanal laser resection?
(No ↓) No clear pattern?	Yes	? Investigate (e.g. MRI scan) ? Rare cause (e.g. thalamic pain) ? Emotional causes • See Pain Problems

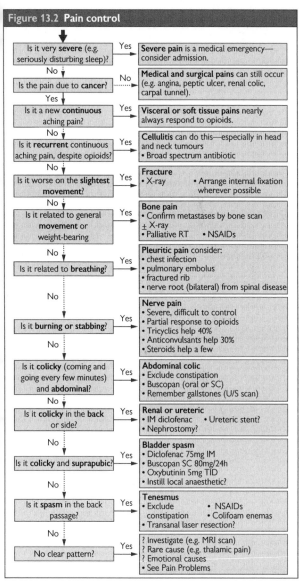

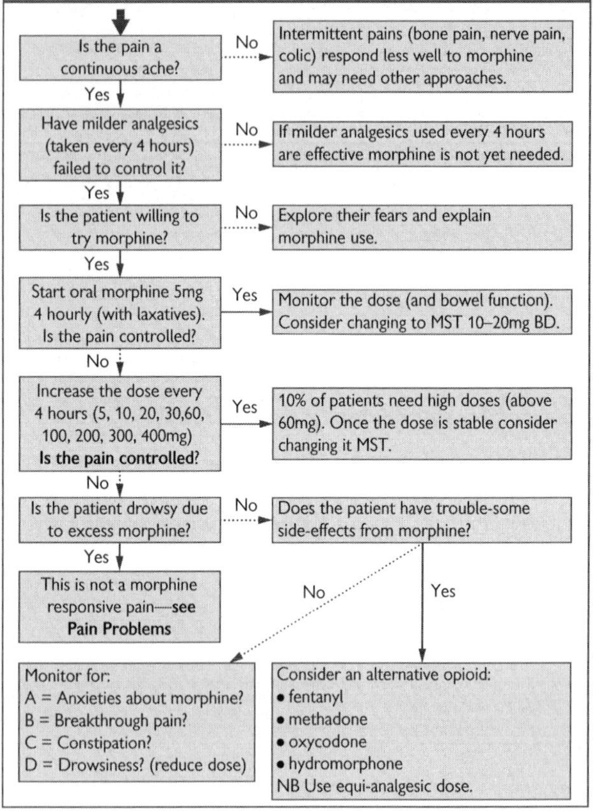
Is the pain a continuous ache?
No
Intermittent pains (bone pain, nerve pain, colic) respond less well to morphine and may need other approaches.
Yes
Have milder analgesics (taken every 4 hours) failed to control it?
No
If milder analgesics used every 4 hours are effective morphine is not yet needed.
Yes
Is the patient willing to try morphine?
No
Explore their fears and explain morphine use.
Yes
Start oral morphine 5mg 4 hourly (with laxatives). Is the pain controlled?
Yes
Monitor the dose (and bowel function). Consider changing to MST 10–20mg BD.
No
Increase the dose every 4 hours (5, 10, 20, 30,60, 100, 200, 300, 400mg) **Is the pain controlled?**
Yes
10% of patients need high doses (above 60mg). Once the dose is stable consider changing it MST.
No
Is the patient drowsy due to excess morphine?
No
Does the patient have trouble-some side-effects from morphine?
Yes
This is not a morphine responsive pain—**see Pain Problems**
No
Yes
Monitor for:
A = Anxieties about morphine?
B = Breakthrough pain?
C = Constipation?
D = Drowsiness? (reduce dose)
Consider an alternative opioid:
• fentanyl
• methadone
• oxycodone
• hydromorphone
NB Use equi-analgesic dose.

Figure 13.3 **Morphine Uasage**

Commencing a person on morphine (and its family including diamorphine and codeine) also needs the health-care professional to bear in mind that the drug has an active metabolite (morphine-6-glucuronide). In renal dysfunction this metabolite can accumulate and result in a greater effect from a given dose (McQuay, 2006), thus care needs to be taken in patients who have renal impairment when it could be that less morphine is needed. In addition, ageing has important effects on how drugs affect the individual since alterations in body composition, metabolic rate and glomerular filtration for example, can affect how the body absorbs, metabolizes and excretes these exogenous chemicals (Sutton *et al.* 2002). It is important to take a careful analgesic history before commencing a patient on morphine since the doses of analgesics previously used, and their effectiveness will give an indication as to the correct starting dose. This can vary from patient to patient. It is also worth remembering that although the 'analgesic ladder' approach outlined by the World Health Organization (1990) originally emphasized the role of morphine, it is now recognized that patients vary greatly in their response to different opioids. Opioid rotation may be necessary to find the drug that maximises benefits and minimises side effects for that individual (Portenoy & Lesage, 1999).

Also, the prevalence of painful comorbidities increases in later life and it is often the case that patients with cancer may be experiencing pain from other causes in addition to the pain related to the cancer. Such comorbidities can increase the incidence of pain among older cancer patients, and the whole pain picture needs to be considered.

If a patient's pain is uncontrolled with a dose of morphine which is causing problematic side effects then measures such as the management of these side effects, reducing the dose of opiate, or rotating to a different opiate, and considering the use of adjuvant drugs or co analgesics may be necessary (Colvin *et al.* 2006). Many patients who have pain which responds poorly to opiates have elements of neuropathic pain, and it can be useful to consider how a patient talks about their pain since this type of pain is often described in the terms shown in Box 13.5.

Box 13.5 Descriptors which may indicate a component of nerve pain

Stabbing; shooting; tingling; burning; prickling; numb; cold; hot; shock-like; pins and needles; possibly sporadic.

Nerve pain, depending upon the cause, can require a different approach than the management of pain from a somatic/nociceptive or visceral origin. Twycross (1997) describes neuropathic pain as that which is associated with the factors outlined in Box 13.6.

Box 13.6 Neuropathic pain associations

- Nerve compression—which may respond to a combination of morphine and a corticosteroid such as dexamethasone.
- Sympathetically maintained pain—which is less common and may require a regional sympathetic nerve block.
- Nerve injury—which is often resistant to morphine and steroids (but can respond to adjuvants, see Table 13.1).

Table 13.1 A four step analgesic ladder for nerve injury pain (Twycross 1997)

Step 1	Step 2	Step 3	Step 4
Tricyclic antidepressant *Or* anticonvulsant	Tricyclic antidepressant *And* anticonvulsant	Class 1 cardiac anti-arrhythmic *Or* ketamine	Spinal analgesia

He also suggests a similar approach to the World Health Organization 3-step analgesic ladder cited above when considering interventions for nerve injury pain, although careful diagnosis is essential before intervention:

Bennett *et al.* (2005) have developed a self report version of the Leeds Assessment of Neuropathic Symptoms and Signs pain scale which may be of help in identifying this type of pain in practice.

13.2 Palliative care

A commonly accepted definition of palliative care is that provided by the World Health Organization (2006), Box 13.7.

Box 13.7 World Health Organiszation definition of palliative care

- Provides relief from pain and other distressing symptoms
- Affirms life and regards dying as a normal process
- Intends neither to hasten nor postpone death
- Integrates the psychological and spiritual aspects of patient care
- Offers a support system to help patients live as actively as possible until death
- Uses a team approach to address the needs of patients and their families, including bereavement counselling if indicated
- Will enhance quality of life, and may also positively influence the course of illness
- Is applicable early in the course of illness in conjunction with other therapies that are intended to prolong life, such as chemotherapy or radiation therapy, and includes those investigations needed to better understand and manage distressing clinical complications

Palliative care developed in response to increasing concerns about the standards of care for dying patients and their families (ten Have & Clark, 2002).The traditional focus for this type of care has been the hospice, and it would appear that those patients who are cared for in a hospice environment receive a high standard of care which meets a range of complex needs (Ellershaw *et al.* 2001). However, there is evidence to suggest that despite the fact that guidelines exist outlining recommendations for best practice (the National Council for Hospice and Specialist Palliative Care Services is one of the principal sources for such documents) there is dissatisfaction with the care given to people in the palliative phase of their illness (National Institute for Clinical Excellence, 2004). This is particularly so since not all patients with life limiting illnesses or indeed with cancer are cared for by hospices. More than half a million people aged 65 or older live in care homes, and substantial numbers of people end their lives in these care settings (Social Care Institute for Excellence (SCIE) 2006). Ellershaw and Coackley (2002) comment that excellence in palliative care is not always well understood or practiced outside of hospice settings. Indeed, older people are reported to have difficulty in accessing good quality palliative care services (Seymour & Clark, 2001), and Lloyd-Williams *et al.* (2005) point out that comorbidity in older patients with cancer further complicates the issue and they state that their own experience is such that if a patient with advanced cancer also has dementia then they are unlikely to be admitted to a specialist palliative care unit.

In addition to the NICE (2004) recommendations concerned with supportive and palliative care for people with cancer, The National Council on Ageing (2002) have published a paper which makes recommendations regarding equality, adequacy and appropriateness of palliative care services for older people, including issues about the place of death. Many studies confirm that most people prefer to die at home (Higginson *et al.* 1998), yet in the UK only a quarter of cancer patients do so. The main reasons for admission to a hospital, hospice or care home are a combination of carer breakdown, poor symptom control and poor communication. In a review of out of hours palliative care in the community Thomas (2001) points to the fact that there is evidence to suggest that the provision of good care at home is more difficult to achieve for patients who are:

- Socially/economically deprived
- Elderly
- Experiencing poor symptom control
- Unable to access 24 hour support
- Female
- Suffering from a chronic illness with an ill defined terminal stage.

13.3 Caring for people at the end of life—the last hours or days of life

The realization that a patient is close to death is very important because it changes decision making and care management. Kaye (1999) points out that as a person enters a terminal phase, aiming to prolong life becomes irrelevant, patient comfort takes priority, and increased support for the family and others who are close is necessary. End-of-life care is an important part of palliative care and usually refers to care at a point where it becomes clear that the patient is in a progressive state of decline and perhaps in their last few days, weeks, or even months of life (Higginson, 1997). In order to care for dying patients it is essential to 'diagnose dying' (Ellershaw & Ward, 2003) but this is something which can be fraught with moral and ethical dilemmas for those involved. Indeed, the care of dying patients, whether it is in a hospice setting or elsewhere raises a range of complex and contentious issues which warrant considered reflection for any health care professional who is working within this context (see ten Have & Clark, 2002).

There have been recent initiatives to transfer the hospice model of care into other care settings and the Liverpool Care Pathway (Ellershaw & Wilkinson, 2003) is an example of this, see Box 13.8. Further details of this integrated care pathway can be accessed at http://www.lcp-mariecurie.org.uk/

Box 13.8 A description of the aims of the Liverpool Care Pathway

- Promote evidence-based practice
- Provide guidelines for end-of-life care
- Improve documentation and communication
- Encourage the practice of pre-emptive prescribing thereby anticipating potential problems
- Enable doctors and nurses to deliver optimum care to patients and their families

This issue is again a complex one since not all older patients who have cancer are dying as a result of the cancer; comorbidity may mean that a patient has a different dying trajectory and may have differing and complex symptom control issues. The impact of the Liverpool Care Pathway is currently being evaluated in practice but methodological difficulties can arise when outcome measures relate to the quality of death, and as yet evidence in support of its efficacy is limited to smaller qualitative studies.

13.4 Conclusions

This chapter has aimed to provide an overview of some of the issues arising from pain management in older people, with a focus on cancer care, palliative care and end-of-life care. It has not been possible to fully explore the complex nature of some of these situations and the decision making inherent within such care delivery. With this in mind, the following websites may provide additional reputable and evidence based information and links to other sites.

Box 13.9

www.jr2.ox.ac.uk/bandolier
Bandolier hosts the Oxford Pain Site and provides valuable evidence based information about palliative and supportive care and pain management.

www.hospice-spc-council.org.uk
The National Council for Hospice and Specialist Palliative Care Services – provides information about palliative care, current news and links to other sites.

www.palliative-medicine.org.uk
The association for Palliative Medicine of Great Britain and Ireland. This site has information on palliative care issues and educational opportunities.

www.palliativedrugs.com
This site provides information for health professionals concerning the use of drugs in palliative care and is produced by Robert Twycross, Andrew Wilcock, and Andrew Dickman.

www.who.int/cancer/palliative/en/
World Health Organisation cancer pages with links to WHO publications and recommended guidelines for practice in cancer and palliative care.

References

Agency for Health Care policy and Research (1994). Clinical Guideline Number 9 AHCPR Publication Number 94-0592. Available at: www.hospicepatients.org/clinicalpracticeguidelines1994.html

Ahmedazi S and Brooks D (1997). Transdermal fentanyl versus sustained release oral morphinein cancer pain: preference, efficacy, and quality of life. The TTS-Fentanyl Comparative Trial Group. *Journal of Pain and Symptom Management*, **16**(3), 141–4.

Bennett M, Smith B, Torrance N, *et al.* (2005). The S-LANSS score for identifying pain of predominantly neuropathic origin: validation for use in clinical and postal research. *Journal of Pain*, **6**(3), 149–58.

Bernabei R, Gambassi G, Lapane K, *et al.* (1998). Management of pain in elderly patientswith cancer. SAGE Study Group. Systematic Assessment of Geriatric Drug Use via Epidemiology. *Journal of American Medical Association*, **279**, 1877–82.

Cleary J and Carbone P (2000). Palliative medicine in the elderly. *Cancer* **80**(7), 1335–47.

Colvin L, Forbes K, Fallon M (2006). ABC of Palliative Care – difficult pain. *British Medical Journal*, **332**, 1081–3.

Department of Health (2000). *The NHS Cancer Plan. A plan for investment. A plan for reform.* Department of Health, London.

Ellershaw JE and Coackley A (2002). An integrated care pathway for the dying. *Geriatric Medicine*, **32**(4), 45–9.

Ellershaw JE, Smith C, Overill S, *et al.* (2001). Care of the dying: Setting standards for symptom control in the last 48 hours of life. *Journal of Pain and Symptom Management*, **21**(1), 12–17.

Ellershaw J and Ward C (2003). Care of the dying patient: the last hours or days of life. *British Medical Journal*, **326**, 30–4.

Ellershaw J and Wilkinson S (eds) (2003). *Care of the Dying. A Pathway to Excellence.* Oxford University Press, Oxford.

Fallon M, Hanks G, and Cherny N (2006). ABC of palliative care. Principles of control of cancer pain. *British Medical Journal*, **332**, 1022–4.

Higginson IJ (1997). Health care needs assessment: Palliative and terminal care. In Stevens A, Raferty J, (eds) *Health Care Needs Assessment.* Second Series. Radcliffe Medical Press, Oxford.

Higginson I, Astin P, and Dolan S (1998). Where do cancer patients die? Ten year trends in the place of death of cancer patients in England. *Palliative Medicine*, **12**(5), 353–63.

Jovicevic-Bekic A (2002). Epidemiology of cancer in the elderly. *Archive of Oncology*, **10**(3), 131.

Kaye P (1999). *Decision Making in Palliative Care.* EPL Publications, Northampton.

Lloyd-Williams M, Payne S, and Dennis M (2005). Specialist palliative care in dementia – patients with dementia are unable to access appropriate palliative care. *British Medical Journal*, **330**, 671–2.

McQuay H (2006). *Pain and its control.* Available at: www.jr2.ox.ac.uk/bandolier/booth/painpag/wisdom/C13.html

National Council on Ageing (2002). *End of Life Issues. Policy Position Paper*, London.

National Institute for Clinical Excellence (2004). *Improving Supportive Care and Palliative Care for Adults with Cancer. The Manual.* National Institute for Clinical Excellence, London.

Portenoy R and Lesage P (1999). Management of cancer pain. *Lancet*, **353**, 1695–700.

Portenoy R, Thaler H, and Kornblith A (1994). Symptom prevalence, characteristics and distress in a cancer population. *Quality of Life Research*, **3**, 183–9.

Seymour J and Clark D (2001). Palliative care and geriatric medicine: shared concerns, shared challenges: *Palliative Medicine*, **15**(4), 269–70.

Social Care Institute for Excellence (2005). *SCIE Research briefing 10: Terminal care in care homes* Available at: www.scie.org.uk/publications/briefings/briefing10/index.asp

Sutton L, Porter L, and Keefe F. (2002). Cancer pain at the end of life: a biopsychosocial perspective. *Pain*, **99**, 5–10.

ten Have H and Clark D (eds) (2002). *The Ethics of Palliative Care*. Open University Press, Buckingham.

Thomas K (2001). *Out-of-hours palliative care in the community*. Macmillan Cancer Relief, London.

Turner NJ, Haward RA, Mulley GP, *et al.* (1999). Cancer in old age—is it inadequately investigated and treated? *British Medical Journal*, **319**, 309–12.

Twycross R (1997). *Symptom Management in Advanced Cancer*. Radcliffe Medical Press, Abingdon.

World Health Organization (1990). *Cancer pain relief and palliative care. Report of a WHO expert committee (World Health Organization Technical Report Series 804)*. World Health Organization, Geneva.

World Health Organization (2006). At www.who.int/cancer/palliative/en/

Zech DF, Grond S, Lynch J, *et al.* (1995). Validation of World Health Organization Guidelines for cancer pain relief: a 10 year prospective study. *Pain* **63**(1), 65–76.

Chapter 14

Nursing care

Dee Burrows

Key points

- Assessment is crucial to effective pain control.
- Nurses should employ comfort care for pain management.
- Non-pharmacological strategies can be effective for acute and chronic pain management.
- Medication must be appropriate and administered as prescribed.
- Service development should follow a systematic approach.

14.1 Introduction

Nurses care for older people in primary, secondary, and independent settings. As discussed in Chapter 1, the incidence and complexity of pain is significant in older people. Common causes include arthritis, metabolic and neurological disorders, heart disease, and aches and pains associated with decreasing mobility. This chapter outlines practical approaches to nursing older people in pain.

14.2 Clinical assessment

Nursing care commences with assessment. The depth of assessment depends upon the care setting and individual's context and goals. Assessment of postoperative pain is likely to focus upon intensity and analgesic effectiveness. Conversely, chronic pain assessment should consider physical, emotional, cognitive and behavioural factors within the personal context. Chapter 2 discusses pain assessment and the different tools available.

14.2.1 Assessment in a postoperative setting

Box 14.1 Case study A: Mr Black

69-year-old Mr Black is increasingly disabled with osteoarthritis. He has been admitted for a knee replacement and is worried about the impact on his active social life.

Important issues for assessment:

- Listening to Mr Black's description of pain (intensity, location, nature) and perception of pain relief.
- Identifying the strategies Mr Black finds helpful (see 14.3.6) and negotiating how these may be supported in hospital.
- Discussing Mr Black's rehabilitation concerns with him and the multi-disciplinary team.

14.2.2 Assessment in a pain clinic

Box 14.2 Case study B: Mrs George

78-year-old Mrs George lives with her husband. She has low back pain, sciatica, and depression. The Consultant in Pain refers her and her husband to the CNS for a trial of electrotherapy and pain management advice.

Important issues for assessment:

- In-depth multidimensional assessment taking account of Mrs George's physical responses, thoughts and feelings about pain, impact on behaviour and functional ability.
- Involving Mr George in the assessment of his wife's pain, the impact on him, their relationship, and quality of life.
- Assessing what strategies Mrs George is already using or is open to learning.

14.2.3 Assessment in a care home

Box 14.3 Case study C: Mrs King

84-years-old Mrs King has moved from her daughter's home to a nearby care home. She has painful peripheral diabetic neuropathy and cognitive impairment following a minor CVA.

Important issues for assessment:

- Welcoming Mrs King to her new home and undertaking the assessment over a number of days.
- Involving Mrs King's daughter and community nurses to gain insight into the impact of pain upon Mrs King.
- Taking account of Mrs King's pain pathology and cognitive impairment (Chapter 3).
- Using a categorical scale or a pain assessment tool designed for people with cognitive impairment (Chapter 2; Mann and Carr, 2006).

14.3 Clinical management

Nursing people with pain involves comfort care, non-pharmacological, and pharmacological approaches. 'Comfort care is the action taken to promote comfort' (Burrows and Baillie, 2005, p507). It is individualized, directed to the whole person, and creative. Successful comfort care leaves the recipient feeling valued and cared for. Strategies include presence, monitoring, touch, comfort talk, and physical actions. Each helps reduce the impact of pain.

14.3.1 Presence

To 'be' with someone with pain can be emotionally draining, leaving nurses and families feeling helpless. Yet 'being there' has been shown to promote comfort and reduce pain (Burrows and Baillie, 2005). Being there for Mrs and Mr George includes involving them both in the consultation, valuing their responses and relationship, supporting Mr George as the primary carer, enabling him to feel less helpless and more able to assist his wife in transferring the strategies the CNS is teaching back to the home environment.

14.3.2 Monitoring

Studies demonstrate that monitoring, described by Hawley (2000) as 'vigilance', is perceived as comforting by patients. Monitoring involves on-going assessment. Nurses may undertake this role or support family doing so. Mr George observed and checked his wife undertaking the taught exercises, relaxation, and pacing towards negotiated goals. The CNS' role was to teach Mr George how to do this, listen to, and record his assessment. Monitoring Mr Black's postoperative pain is an important aspect of postoperative recovery. Competent and confident assessments have the potential to inspire confidence, such that Mr Black should be more able to hear, internalize, and act upon advice regarding the integration of his rehabilitation and social life.

14.3.3 Touch

There are two types of touch: instrumental and expressive. The former is used when undertaking nursing actions, the latter when the intention is to provide comfort. Comforting touch must be used consciously and intentionally (Moore and Gilbert, 1995). Nurses must be sensitive to recipients' responses as cultural and individual significance to touch varies. Touch—touching hands, stroking, patting, rocking, holding—can be calming, promote relaxation, the production of endorphins, and compete with pain stimuli at the 'gate'. Mr Black may appreciate a confident touch on his arm offering reassurance as the nurse helps him out of bed during the first few postoperative days. Mrs King may find stroking comforting, though care must be taken with the location as neuropathic pain can result in touch being interpreted as pain (allodynia). Alternatively connecting touch—a brief light touch—as the nurse enters or leaves Mrs King's room may provide comfort.

14.3.4 Comfort talk

Hawley (2000) identified four types of comforting talk: reassuring ('don't worry, I'm here'); coaching (helping people stay in control and cope); explanatory (providing information, responding to questions); and empathetic (conveying understanding and caring). Comfort talk helps people to endure situations (Morse and Proctor, 1998)—such as pain—and communicates caring. It is carried out face-to-face, often in a slow, rhythmic manner and with good eye contact. CPM (continuous passive motion) machines are frequently employed following knee replacements to help patients recover their range of knee movement. Because of oedema and pain, patients find the treatment uncomfortable. Explaining the purpose of CPM to Mr Black, reassuring him that it will get better, empathising that it is a challenging part of postoperative recovery, and coaching to take regular analgesics and use relaxation while undergoing CPM can help reduce discomfort. Mrs George may find that comfort talk helps her focus, despite her depression, and thus learn new skills to cope with her pain. Comfort talk is a particularly useful strategy for Mrs King given the complexity of her physical and cognitive situation.

14.3.5 Physical actions

Comfort and pain relief can also be achieved through positioning and posture management while the person is seated or in bed; ensuring mattresses are comfortable and bedding appropriate; assisting with hygiene, elimination, and nutrition. Actions need to be thought through and combined with other comfort care approaches if the person is to feel actively cared for rather than simply physically comfortable and pain free (Tutton and Seers, 2004). On initial assessment, Mrs George described how her back pain interfered with sleep. The

CNS suggested she try a duvet under the bottom sheet as a mattress topper. The ensuing increase in comfort reduced Mrs George's night time pain and improved her sleep.

14.3.6 **Non-pharmacological management**

Non-pharmacological management includes self-generated, taught, technical, and alternative strategies (see Chapter 11 for the latter). Self generated and taught strategies are well integrated into chronic pain management where evidence for effectiveness exists. They are less will addressed in acute care. However, Burrows (2000) found that identifying and supporting orthopaedic patients' self-generated strategies reduced postoperative anxiety, opioid consumption, pain and distress.

- **Distraction** involves concentrating on something other than the pain. It can increase perceptions of control and help reduce pain intensity and impact for brief periods, e.g. watching TV, reading, listening to music, socializing, and hobbies. Nurses must be aware that just because someone is engaged in one of these activities, does not mean they are pain-free. The nurse could encourage Mr Black to invite his friends to visit and Mrs King to socialize with other residents. Mrs George was encouraged to resume knitting, which she had previously undertaken as a hobby and distraction from pain.
- **Relaxation** reduces muscle tension, mental distress, anxiety, and fatigue promoting calmness, and sleep (Nicholas *et al.* 2003). Various short and long techniques are used for mild to moderate pain, including breathing, progressive muscular techniques and imagery. The latter involves imaging sights, sounds, odours, taste and touch, for example a stroll through a garden on a warm summer's day. In Burrows' (2000) study, patients were asked to describe their technique to the nurse so they could be talked through them when drowsy, awaiting analgesics, or mobilizing postoperatively. Mr Black was supported in this way, while Mrs George was taught emergency and short techniques, practising them with her husband. Mrs King was taught a longer relaxation to use when her daughter was leaving to minimize distress.
- **Warmth and cold** are useful pain management techniques. Wheat packs, heat pads, and wraps are widely available, reduce muscle tension and enhance blood flow, comfort, and analgesia. Cold packs and ice help reduce inflammatory pain. They should not be used over wounds, as cold decreases healing rates. Some people prefer either heat or cold and their preferences should be considered. Physiotherapists are a useful resource in determining whether heat, cold, or a combination is appropriate.

- **Exercise** eases muscle stiffness and tension, promotes fitness and has the potential to reduce pain (Chapter 12). The nurses' role is usually to support and encourage the person to maintain exercises prescribed by the physiotherapist. They may also advise on the integration of exercise into daily activities. For example, Mrs George was encouraged to undertake gentle exercises each time she waited for the kettle to boil. Mrs King was reminded to do five minutes of chair exercise when given her medication just before meals.
- **Trancutaneous electrical nerve stimulation (TENS) and trancutaneous spinal electroanalgesia (TSE)** are 'technical' ways of treating pain. The devices deliver short electrical pulses through the skin to peripheral nerves (TENS) or the spinal cord (TSE). Treatments can be self-managed or nurse administered. Training is needed to get the best effects. Mrs George underwent a trial of both with the CNS.
- **Cognitive behavioural therapy** (CBT) is discussed in Chapter 9. CBT takes account of the interplay between physical responses to pain, thoughts, feelings, associated behaviour, and the individual's personal context. Nurses trained in using cognitive behavioural principles are able to employ these in assisting people to manage persistent pain. Referral for CBT should be considered for older people, including Care Home residents (The Australian Pain Society, 2005).

14.3.7 **Medication management**

Important principles for medication management:

- General knowledge of pharmacokinetic and pharmacodynamic age-related changes (Chapter 7; Mann and Carr, 2006).
- Older people may have reduced sensitivity to mild and moderate pain for which simple analgesics combined with comfort and non-pharmacological strategies can be effective.
- Studies indicate an age-related decline in tolerating severe or persistent pain (Gibson, 2006).
- Increased sensitivity to opioids should be acknowledged in the dose and frequency of administration, rather than be regarded as rationale for not using opioids with older persons.
- Knowledge of the reduced margin between toxic and therapeutic doses should guide practice in administering NSAIDs (Seers, 2003).
- Nurses administering prescribed combinations of analgesics, NSAIDs and/or drugs for neuropathic pain (e.g. antidepressants and anticonvulsants) must observe and monitor effect carefully, be aware of side effect profiles and seek medical consultation as appropriate. This caveat applies equally to the three case studies.

- Gibson (2006) highlights that the typical 70-year-old living at home has at least three comorbid health problems and takes on average seven different medications daily. Mrs King may be taking insulin, antihypertensives, a statin, analgesics, and medication for neuropathic pain concurrently. Understanding drug interactions is paramount to safe practice.
- Nurses must ensure that older people with pain (and their carers) understand their medication (purpose, effects, side effects, and administration) if confusion and non-compliance are to be minimized (Scholfield *et al.* 2005). Mr Black is likely to be discharged on analgesics and needs to know how to balance rehabilitation with a gradual reduction in medication; Mrs and Mr George need to know when she should take her pain medication and anti-depressants to minimize side effects and maximize effect; while Mrs King needs to know what her medication is for each time it is administered.
- CNS may consider liaison with local Care Homes where social care staff are frequently responsible for medication administration.
- Keeping up-to-date and following local practice guidelines are essential for safe effective medication management of pain.

14.4 Developing your service—reflection points

Quality nursing care is dependent not simply upon knowing how to assess and manage an individual's pain, but also upon critical self-reflection and service development. The framework presented below contains a number of questions that can be used as prompts when considering how to develop services for older people with pain and the clinical practice guidelines you need. The questions should be addressed in order as each may require a sequence of discussions and actions before you can move on to the next step.

Box 14.4 What is your vision for older people with pain?

You might consider discussing this within the team and with patients, residents, and carers. What is it you are trying to achieve? How does this fit with the setting philosophy? Are you focusing on care, training and education, management and resources, or a combination of these?

Box 14.5 What are your goals?

The discussions will help you to identify the areas that you want to focus on. You may then need to prioritize. Having decided the aspect that you want to start with, you then need to identify your end goal/s. This is important if you are to develop the service and/or yourself in a systematic way and know when you have achieved your goals.

Box 14.6 What is your current approach?

Remember that there will be much in your current practice that is already excellent. With your goals in mind, consider what your current approach can bring to your new goal/s.

Box 14.7 How did you arrive at it?

Your current approach was developed for a reason. What was that reason? Asking yourself this question will help you to check that your new vision is compatible with your setting and any pertinent national directives. It will also highlight any barriers and opportunities there are in moving forward.

Box 14.8 What are the alternative ways to moving towards your new goal?

There is always more than one way to achieve a goal. You need to consider alternatives and the advantages and disadvantages of each It is possible that your favoured approach is not as practical and realistic as you first thought. A less favoured approach may actually help you to achieve your goal and vision more effectively and speedily.

Box 14.9 What is your action plan—to get from where you are now to where you want to be?

Consider the steps that you need to take. Are there implications for training and education, resources, communication, patient and carer involvement? Who will lead on each step and what is the timetable? What support does the leader need?

Box 14.10 How will you know when you are there?

You need to know that each step is completed before moving on. You also need to know when you have reached your end goal and to ensure that it still fits with your vision. Check back, ask yourself these questions, and congratulate yourself on the achievements. You may now decide to start addressing your second goal. Do not forget to maintain the new developments achieved through working to the first goal.

You may want to look at published guidelines for managing pain in older people and some useful ones are provided in the references.

In addition, the recently published survey by The Patients Association (The Patients Association, 2007) illuminates the challenges and offers some ideas for service development.

14.5 Conclusions

Nursing older people in pain can be both challenging and rewarding. Assessment is crucial to achieving effective pain control. Pain management should focus on older peoples' needs and preferences, using comfort care, non-pharmacological strategies, and appropriate medication. Adopting a sequential framework can help facilitate personal and service development. In combination, these are vital if the pain experienced by older people is to be effectively managed.

References

Burrows D (2000). *Engaging Patients in Their own Pain Management.* Unpublished PhD Thesis. Brunel University.

Burrows D and Bailie L (2005). Managing pain and promoting comfort. In Baillie L (ed). *Developing Practical Nursing Skills.* 2nd ed. pp.485–522.

Gibson S (2006). Older people's pain. *Pain Clinical Updates*, **XIV**, No. 3, June.

Hawley MP (2000). Nurse comforting strategies: perceptions of emergency department patients. *Clinical Nursing Research*, **9**, 441–59.

Mann E and Carr E (2006) *Pain Management: Essential Clinical Skills for Nurses.* Blackwell Publishing, Oxford.

Moore JR and Gilbert DA (1995). Elderly residents: perceptions of nurses' comforting touch. *Journal of Gerontological Nursing*, **21**, 6–13.

Morse JM and Proctor A (1998). Maintaining patient endurance: the comfort work of trauma nurses. *Clinical Nursing Research*, **7**, 250–74.

Nicholas M, Molloy A, Tonkin L *et al.* (2003). *Manage Your Pain.* Souvenir Press, London.

Seers K (2003). Pain and older people. In Redfern SJ and Ross FM (eds.) *Nursing Older People* 3rd ed. Churchill Livingstone, Edinburgh.

Schofield P, Dunham M, and Black C (2005). *Older People—Managing Their Pain in the Community Setting.* www.jcn.co.uk/journal.asp?monthnum=09&yearnum=2005&type=search&articleid=844

The Australian Pain Society (2005). *Pain in Residential Aged Care Facilities: Management Strategies.* www.apsoc.org.au

The Patients Association (2007). Pain in Older People; A Hidden Problem. www.patients-association.org.uk/news_level2.asp?level2_ID=467, accessed 27th March 2007.

Tutton E and Seers K (2004). Comfort on a ward for older people. *Journal of Advanced Nursing*, **46**(4), 380–9.

Useful web addresses

Epidemiology

www.arthritis.org
www.arthritiscare.org.uk
www.boneandjointdecade.org
www.cdc.gov
www.iasp-pain.org

Osteoporosis

www.nice.org.uk/download.aspx?o=TA087quickrefguide
www.csp.org.uk/uploads/documents/OSTEOgl.pdf
www.nos.org.uk/search-results/coping-with-pain.htm&pm=
scch_EF1182BF67123DE2A858059590796E22

Pain and addiction

http://www.foresight.gov.uk/
http://www.samhsa.gov/

Occupational and physiotherapy

http://www.nelh.nhs.uk/cochrane.asp
http://www.cot.org.uk/members/publications/free/briefings/pdf/
23Definitions&CoreSkills.pdf
http://www.pedro.fhs.usyd.edu.au/index.html

Palliative care, cancer care, and end of life

www.jr2.ox.ac.uk/bandolier
www.hospice-spc-council.org.uk
www.palliative-medicine.org.uk
www.palliativedrugs.com
This site provides information for health professionals concerning the use of drugs in www.who.int/cancer/palliative/en/
www.ncpc.org.uk
www.hospicepatients.org/clinicalpracticeguidelines1994.html

Nursing care

The American Geriatrics Society: www.americangeriatrics.org
The American Pain Society: www.ampainsoc.org
The Australian Pain Society: www.apsoc.org.au
The British Pain Society: www.britishpainsociety.org

Index

B

C

D

E

F

G

H

Printed and bound by CPI Group (UK) Ltd, Croydon, CR0 4YY